First Edition

ISBN-13 978-0692615706
ISBN-10 0692615709

Cultivating Science & Weeding Out Lore:
Medical Cannabis in Pediatric Neurology and Palliative Care

✳

A practical primer for parents and providers.

Marie-Helene B. Grzesiak
with Laura Bultman, MD (ed.)

Wrenchworks Reference Library Press
Minneapolis, MN

For Matthew and Eleanor
who continue to prove everyone wrong, defy the odds,
and baffle medical science at every turn.

❋

❧Table of Contents❧

DISCLAIMER: *The information provided in this book is not intended to be a comprehensive review of the literature nor is it a substitute for medical education, medical or legal advice. Medical cannabis research is a quickly evolving field, and cannabis laws are rapidly changing. Stay informed.*

≀ *Foreword* ≀

A quick, simple, and painfully honest medical cannabis reference guide for parents, caregivers and health care providers of children with neurological, degenerative or terminal disorders and diagnoses... It seemed like a straightforward, albeit heart-wrenching request at the onset.

As a writer, educator and science communicator, I've been involved in the review, analysis and dissemination of information regarding medical cannabis and its potential for use in pediatric neuropalliative care for some time. A few months ago, parents and health care providers started approaching me to ask if I'd be willing to provide them with a missing tool for their toolbox. The message was universal: *We'd like answers to our questions. We'd like information we can trust. We'd like it all in one place. We'd like a book that covers the basics and bridges the understanding gaps between science, lore, expectations and reality. Wouldn't hurt if it could make us laugh in the process*[1].

I made a few calls, organized a few meetings, raided a few libraries and piles of newly released journals and papers. I leveraged the contacts I'd made in the

---

1 Because of this request for humor to lighten difficult topics, this book almost ended up titled "Potholes: The bumpy road to medical cannabis for pediatric palliative care." *Almost.*

medical cannabis, pediatric neurology, and palliative care worlds. I girded my loins – there are instructions online, for the curious, should you need to gird yours someday – and I agreed to give it a go.

I had multiple dogs in this race: at the forefront of my mind, my own child, who struggled with a unique variant of a rare neurological disorder, and who might be helped by medical cannabis. Also in my mind were my fellow parents, who struggle to separate the snake-oil salesmen from the people who are genuinely trying to help. And finally, my fellow scientists who need synthesized, condensed, quick-reference information, and who have vowed to *first do no harm.*

This book came together with the help of a group of people who understand that this painful quest for the big hope that comes from such a small plant is one that requires several moving parts. It requires cooperation, dedication, and the understanding that fundamentally, patients and their families have a right to take risks, no matter how big, no matter how small. *It also requires open minds and a healthy dose of pragmatism.*

It's a tough garden to tend to, as it requires putting aside a natural tendency towards distrust and reservation. We are not unlike settlers in a frozen wasteland: the only way to survive and thrive in the harsh conditions will be to help each other reach a common goal – easing the suffering of these children in our care.

There are no guarantees. There aren't even promises. What there is, however, is hope. Big hope with reservation and caution, but big hope all the same.

My journey through this, as a pragmatist and as a parent, has taught me that the camps most commonly involved represent a wealth of *good people doing good work for the sake of people in need.*

For parents and caregivers

This guide is here to walk you through the process, to help you talk intelligently and efficiently about these possibilities with your loved one's healthcare provider. It will help you sort out what is rooted in sound science versus cannabis lore, and to help you approach the possibilities with as many facts as we currently have.

Things change rapidly at times, especially from a legal standpoint, at both the federal and the state level. Research is changing our understanding of things, too. It is becoming harder and harder to keep up with progress for those in the field, let alone for medical professionals and invested parents who have children to care for and households to run.

Don't rely on what you read on message boards online, or from potentially unreliable advocacy news sources. Beware politically charged websites. Pay close attention to the dates on any publication or posting: this is a field where information becomes outdated quickly.

When in doubt, talk to the staff at your dispensary. Make sure they have the appropriate credentials and education. Talk to your healthcare providers, if they're in the know. Talk to your manufacturer or distributor's staff pharmacist and staff medical directors (who are hopefully medical doctors). Talk to your state's medical cannabis office about regulations and updates.

Look for rational, calm, pragmatic advocacy groups in your area who are looking to make changes *that are pertinent to you and your family,* one step at a time, and who have good working relationships with your state's manufacturers. Reach out to other parents. Reach out to medical professionals.

Keep your wits about you.

Remember the following, as a bit of a mission statement:

> *This journey isn't about cure and recovery – it's about incremental relief*
> *of symptoms, quality of life, and about*
> *making the whole picture better than it was before.*

For medical professionals

As interest in medical cannabis and, more specifically, in *cannabinoids* in their isolated forms has exploded onto the research scene, the publication of research materials has been outpacing our ability to keep up with the influx of new data. There aren't enough hours in the day, between patient caseloads and notes, meetings, teaching and mentoring, rounds and conferences to read *everything*. Especially not when the number of papers on the topic, in peer-reviewed journals, is growing faster than we ever anticipated. Trying to sort out where to start, who to trust, and how to prioritize investigation time into cannabinoid research is enough to drive anyone to distraction.

Despite knowing that change is coming, that the political tides are changing, and that the pool of data is growing, cannabis research in the United States is *relatively* new. A lot of our collective knowledge has been heavily influenced by *cannabis lore*, the war on drugs, and the addiction discourse. As scientists, we owe it to ourselves to remain pragmatic until we hold data that proves efficacy in our hot little hands. But as piles upon piles of well-documented case studies reach our desks, it becomes harder to ignore.

You may find yourself in a position where your drive to help your patients and their families is at odds with your professional need for years of double-blind clinical studies to back up a course of treatment. One of the greatest challenges physicians face is bridging the chasm between disease pathology and illness experience: you can be authoritative about the first, but not about the second. Respecting the latter can help guide both medical and ethical decisions in the treatment of your young patients.

Intractability[2] proves to be another considerable challenge. Mathematicians and physicians seem to share a similar itch when it comes to intractable problems: these problems can be solved in *theory*, given enough time and infinite means, but in practice, finding a solution to them takes too long for their solutions to be useful. By its definition, hardwired in our brains, *intractable problems and intractable disorders are too complex, difficult to change, manipulate, or resolve.* Therein lies the greatest enemy of the neuropalliative care patient: *inertia*. This intractability problem stops us dead in our tracks and, sometimes, discourages us to the point of abandoning attempts at searching for solutions.

Quickly, all that is *intractable* lands in the lap of the palliative care specialists, since no one else wants to deal with things that can't be fixed. What happens when we discover *something* that might prove helpful in taking a bite out of an *intractable* disorder? Patients, parents and caregivers are overwhelmed with information (both good and bad).

These patients and their families are vulnerable to the siren song of cures and panaceas, and to snake oil salesmen who lurk in the dark corners feasting on despair, waiting to pounce and make a tidy profit in the process. And physicians try to reconcile new data (that no one has time to sift through) with the nature of intractability, disease pathology, and patient illness experience. What's a physician to do?

This guide is here to walk you through the current status of medical cannabis and its use in pediatric palliative care, its promises and its pitfalls, and help illuminate the path a little by shining light on both the forest and the trees. Just

---

2 *Intractability* is defined as being *resistant to treatment*.

like parents and caregivers, physicians are *not alone* walking down this new path. There are fellow physicians and scientists out there who are willing and able to accompany you and your patients on the journey.

The organization of this book relies heavily on a modified Socratic or dialectic method to approach material, answering common questions asked by parents and providers alike in an approachable but scientifically complete and accurate way. An emphasis has been put on pragmatism and modest expectations, as well as on the importance of cooperation between families, dispensary staff, and medical teams in order to provide the best care possible.

For families outside the United States

The information contained in this book will hopefully be helpful to you in your journey, as it is, on the whole, not geopolitically bound. The legal challenges faced by American families may be similar to those you face in your jurisdiction, or may bring to light potential issues you might face and give you food for thought. Some countries have slowly been embracing the potential of medical cannabis, legally, thanks to the power of the population pushing for legal changes despite strong political opposition.

As always, legal and medical information changes quickly. Keep an eye out for changing legislation, and an ear to the ground for laws challenging the use of medical cannabis in pediatrics in particular. Get involved. And, when in doubt, always consult the proper authorities in your country.

International cooperation, and the genesis of this book

Some of the most helpful medical cannabis communities have been run by parents who collaborate across borders and over oceans, online. They have formed communities around pediatric use of medical cannabis (sometimes with condition-specific subgroups) rather than politics. These parents were among those who gave a huge push for this book to be published and I am forever grateful for their support, motivation, and encouragement. May we finally have a repository of information that is easy to access, for all.

Special thanks

Many thanks to my little one's core team of tireless professionals -Tim, John, Scott, Daniel, Kelli, Jennifer, Britta - without whom the world would have continued to be a confusing maelstrom of sound and fury, for all they've done and all they continue to do.

Hat tip to my fellow parents-on-the-hills, who have fought hard to get to where we are today. I have learned so much from you, and continue to do so, every day. Paige, an inspiration, always. Annette, for the sporks. Angie, Kathy, Kimberly, Patrick, Michelle and Jai for their fearless trailblazing.

Editorial and professional nods to Kevin Kulp, for donning the muse robes; to Julie O'Connor at Wrenchworks, for all she does; to Sara Cooper, who keeps me sane, catches my stray commas, and edits like the wind; to Martin Kilmer, for embracing the madness, all those years ago; and to Kari and Christine for the countless rescues from being trapped between the doors out front at MinnMed. And to rest of the gang: Kyle, Amber, Karen, and Ross, for humoring me.

Joe, for always being there.

And of course Dr. Laura Bultman, best editor and collaborator a writer could ask for, for keeping the noodles crispy, the coffee flowing, and the neurons firing.

~M.-H. B. Grzesiak
January 2016

❧ I ❧

Introduction to Medical Cannabis in Pediatric Neurology and Neuropalliative Care: Promises and Pitfalls

anacea was the Greek goddess of universal remedy who walked the Earth with a potion that had the power to cure the sick and heal the wounded. She and most of her divine siblings shared similar talents. Her sisters Hygieia, Iaso and Aceso looked over matters of cleanliness and sanitation, recuperation and the healing process. Two of her brothers were equally gifted: Podaleirius as a diagnostician, and Machaon as a master surgeon.

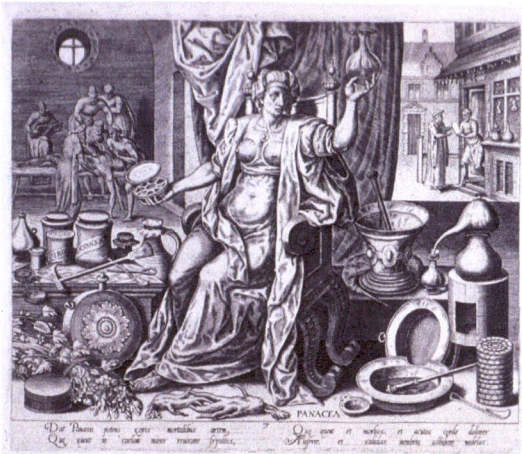

Illustration 1: "Panacea." Engraving, 19 x 25 cm, National Library of Medicine's History of Medicine Collection. Public Domain.

We have been seeking Panacea's potion for centuries. Most of the time, our motives for doing so are noble. *Human beings seem to have an innate drive to better the lives of their fellow man and ease his suffering.* This isn't to say that the quest for bettering our fellow man's circumstances hasn't been motivated by greed and self-importance at times. On the whole, however, we are a compassionate species, and many dedicate their lives to better the lives of others.

When it comes to children and adults with incurable diseases and syndromes that rob them of their quality of life, desperation, frustration and sheer exhaustion lead us to seek a cure-all. A Panacea – both the goddess and her cure. We wish it so much that sometimes we try to will one into existence.

If you are reading this book, it is likely that your profession as a compassionate health care provider, caregiver or worker in another official or political capacity has led you down this road. It is also possible that you've been thrown onto this path through life's complex and painful twists and turns, in the hopes of easing a loved one's suffering.

Whether you are approaching medical cannabis with extreme caution or wild abandon, the path isn't completely dark, and full of both promises and pitfalls.

※ ※ ※

Cannabis has long been thought of as a panacea. It's not the only plant to have had this reputation. In the past, we thought this of foxglove, rosy periwinkle, and poppy. These three plants have wonderful medical applications today, but none are *panaceas*. All are potent *medicines* when made and administered in controlled conditions and for appropriate conditions. There is no reason to believe that the same couldn't true of cannabis. Like any other substance, it has the potential to cause benefit or harm, depending on how it is used, and who uses it.

Movie tropes lead us all to crave magical antidotes, cures to medical conditions that will be a fix to the things that ail us. With the exception of a handful of scenarios, the truth is that most medical conditions have no *cure*. Medical conditions can be *treated and managed.* They require daily maintenance, which might include daily medications for example. No matter what, it requires work and monitoring.

We have all seen, read, or heard stories of near-miraculous recoveries or astounding improvement involving children and medical cannabis. These stories are true, however they are the stories of the *outliers* – the statistical anomalies who respond in extraordinary ways to cannabinoids. We are learning more and more about these remarkable children as science marches on, and we hope to harness the secrets of their unusual success someday.

Before engaging on this journey, it is best to keep your expectations modest and realistic. Don't lose sight of the reason you want to try medical cannabis in the first place: It's about incremental relief and better quality of life, not about complete recovery or cure.

Cannabis has immense potential. As parents, we need to think of it in terms of *improving quality of life* and in terms of palliative management of our children's complex medical conditions. If we can reduce their painful, life-endangering, consciousness-robbing symptoms even by a little, why not try?

However, if we do try, we need to proceed with knowledge, caution, and level-headedness. Do not fall into the Great Panacea Trap. There lies madness. We need to be naturally wary of any medicine that purports to cure *everything*. As we go down this path, parents and medical professionals need to keep the following four points in mind:

---

1 *Do no harm.*
2 *Set pragmatic goals.*
3 *Improve quality of life by reducing troublesome symptoms and negative drug side-effects.*
4 *Anything above and beyond that is a fringe benefit.*

Panaceas come and go, with extraordinary claims but little to no peer-reviewed, carefully studied evidence to back up those claims. Medical cannabis has recently seen an important and steady increase in peer-reviewed research. Currently, every week, there's an average of fourteen new scientific publications on the topic. We're understanding more about it, and we're studying medical cannabis and its components in greater depth.

We've discovered that the *active constituents* of cannabis – closely related compounds called *cannabinoids* – do have the power to help a with a number of conditions. The search for answers has led scientists to an important discovery – the endocannabinoid system – a unique communication system in the brain and body that affects important functions like appetite, pain modulation, sleep, stress response, and memory.

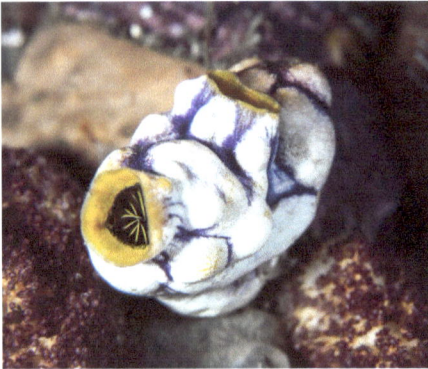

Illustration 2: Who's got an endocannabinoid system, just like we humans do? This handsome guy. Colorful Tunicate [sea squirt] on Coral Reef. Getty Images.

In the word *endocannabinoid,* it's the *endo-* prefix that should catch your attention. It stands for *endogenous.* Humans and other critters come standard with one of these systems[3]. *Practical!*

The endocannabinoid system has been studied through genetic and pharmacological methods – the only way to do so legally until very recently. Roundworms (and other nematodes), sea squirts and all vertebrates including humans have an endocannabinoid system, and by comparing the genetics of the cannabinoid receptors in different species, it's now thought that the endocannabinoid system has been around for over 600 million years.

---

3   Does this remind you of endorphins ("endo-morphine"), chemicals found in poppies, and our pre-wired system meant to handle opiates? It should.

Endocannabinoid molecules, which are found in the nervous systems of humans and other animals, share chemical similarities with compounds found in cannabis. In the 1990s, five endocannabinoids were identified, but two emerged as being particularly important: anandamide (AEA) and 2-arachidonoylglycerol (2-AG). All five are linked by one common root – arachidonic acid – a fatty acid similar to omega-6 fatty acids.

Endocannabinoids aren't classic neurotransmitters in that they aren't stored the same way, and they are produced on demand in response to injury[4].   When endocannabinoids are produced in our bodies, they stimulate cannabinoid receptors. They act locally on cannabinoid receptors, and are immediately metabolized after their action.

There are at least two types of these cannabinoid receptors. The most well-known and well-studied are CB1 and CB2, which serve distinct functions in our well being:

> *CB1 receptors* are found mostly in the brain, spinal cord and other parts of the body including the heart, retina, uterus, testes, liver, small intestine and peripheral nerve cells.

> *CB2 receptors* are found mostly on cells of the immune system (including the spleen), T-cells, B-cells and macrophages, as well as bone cells.

Cannabinoids bind to these receptors, interacting with them similarly to the way a key fits into a lock. If we imagine the cannabinoid key attaching itself to its receptor lock in a cell wall, an effect is unlocked on the brain and in the body.

The way cannabinoids and endocannabinoids act upon the brain is no longer as mysterious as it once was. For example, in 2002, Marsiacano and his team of researchers published an article in the journal *Nature* identifying a key clinical

---

4   Injury is used, here, in its broadest medical sense.

downstream effect: Marsiacano successfully demonstrated that the endocannabinoid system could control the extinction of aversive memories in people with post-traumatic stress disorder. When cannabinoids bind to the receptor cells of the amygdala, they appear to have a direct effect on brain function and the minimization of aversive memories.

Along the same lines, scientists have been able to show, through animal and bench research models, that a number of cannabinoid actions are mediated via CB1 and/or CB2 receptors. We now know, for example, that CB1 is involved in receptor-mediated modulation of epileptiform and seizure activity. We have also discovered that these receptors are not the only mechanisms at play in the modulation of seizure activity.

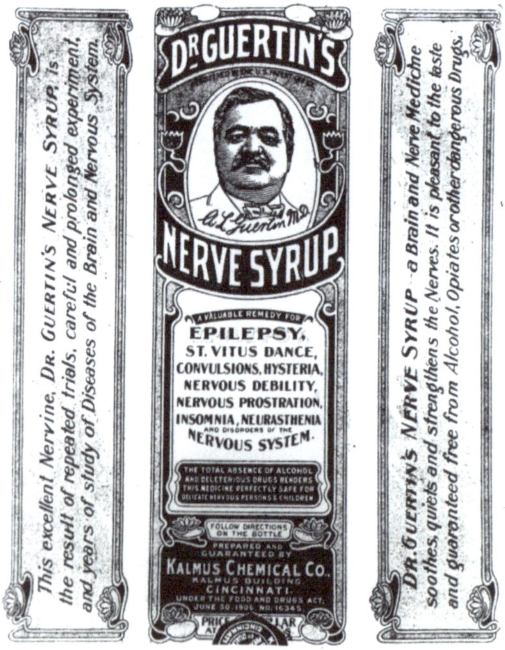

Illustration 3: "Dr. Guertin's nerve syrup" (191?), 9 x 7cm photomechanical print, National Library of Medicine's History of Medicine Collection. Public Domain.

Author's note:

A small digression in the form of a sidebar – Scientists now more than ever before have reason to believe that cannabis medicine isn't just a grab bag of lore, nostrums and quackery.

Let us take a moment to banish the ads for *Dr. Guertin's Nerve Syrup* and other such potions from the 1900s from our collective memories.

Right.

Carry on.

The most popular cannabinoid for the treatment of intractable epilepsies in children, cannabidiol (CBD), shows only a negligible affinity for CB1 and CB2 receptors. It's possible that the anti-convulsant effects of CBD are due to a receptor-independent mechanism that we are only now starting to uncover.

Other research has uncovered that anandamide and 2-AG's activation of CB1 and/or CB2 can have quite extensive local effects. They include (but aren't limited to) effects involving myocardial contractility, platelet activation, endothelial cell activation, adhesion of inflammatory cells, neutrophil activation, monocyte recruitment and transmigration, release of inflammatory cytokines, T-cell recruitment and activation, protection against ischemic injuries (CB2), reduction in blood pressure (CB1), anti-arrhythmic action (CB1), reduction of shock episodes (both CB1 and CB2) and anti-atherogenic activity (CB2).

It's been difficult to find out how the human body is *already built* to process cannabinoids (much like we are built to process *opioids*) and how we can harness it to help ease the suffering of patients because it's been nearly universally illegal – or practically impossible – to conduct research into the matter until very recently. Fortunately, animal studies and bench science have been able to elucidate basic mechanisms.

We know a lot, but we have much to learn. What we do know, however, is that no matter how promising medical treatment with cannabis might be, and how fascinating our endocannabinoid system is, medical cannabis is not a panacea.

Seeing beyond the panacea: Cultivating science

Medical cannabis can be considered a potential neuropalliative treatment approach for a variety of conditions where other treatment methods have failed. It is important *not* to assume that it is a replacement for other treatment modalities. It is *best used as an* adjunctive[5] *in almost all cases, rather than as* monotherapy.

> The word *palliative* tends to strike fear in the heart of parents because we associate it with end of life care. While the term can rightfully be associated with hospice care, *palliative care* simply means treatment that is meant to *alleviate symptoms* of an underlying incurable condition without the intent to treat its root cause. In other words, the treatment itself isn't aiming to *cure. It's aiming to make life better by relieving symptoms of the underlying condition.*

The field of pediatric oncology has been hit particularly hard by the *cannabis panacea pitfall.* When it comes to the treatment of pediatric cancers – especially those with poor prognosis – it becomes difficult not to be lured by promises of cures and miracles. The cannabis industry has certainly made these claims over the years, and it is possible that some patients have made recoveries. Statistical anomalies do not a cure or a cancer panacea make. *Do not forego conventional treatment for the siren song of unproven claims.*

The same type of *cure* promises have cropped up in the treatment of seizure disorders, preying on parents and caregivers in desperate need of hope. Keep expectations modest, and keep an open mind regarding adjunctive versus monotherapeutic use of medical cannabis.

Above all else, don't lose sight of the goals of reducing and relieving symptoms, and bettering quality of life.

---

5 Added to, supplementary to other medications, working on concert with other medications, rather than as a single agent.

Cannabis has had a long track record of being helpful with a wide number of conditions that fall into the neuropalliative category, as well as a number of others including, but not limited to[6]:

- ✔ seizure disorders
- ✔ Tourette syndrome and neurological tics
- ✔ intractable muscle spasms, such as those experienced in multiple sclerosis and cerebral palsy, spinal cord and nerve injuries
- ✔ intractable pain
- ✔ intractable nausea and severe wasting as seen in cancer
- ✔ HIV, AIDS and AIDS-related disorders
- ✔ Amyotrophic Lateral Sclerosis (ALS / Lou Gehrig's disease)
- ✔ inflammatory bowel disease
- ✔ Alzheimer's disease
- ✔ Huntington's disease
- ✔ hepatitis C
- ✔ glaucoma
- ✔ diabetes
- ✔ arthritis
- ✔ osteoporosis
- ✔ terminal illness and palliative care
- ✔ some psychiatric conditions, including schizophrenia, PTSD and autism

It is important to note that each and every one of these conditions respond differently to different components of cannabis (such as THC or CBD) as part of their treatment.

---

6 Some states may not recognize all of these conditions for the certification of patients under their medical cannabis programs. Some states, such as Minnesota and New York, only recognize a small but growing number of conditions and illnesses, and under very strict definitions and specific circumstances. Other states restrict medical cannabis to oils that contain CBD only, or CBD with 0.3% THC or less. Always keep up to date with your state laws and statutes, which are usually readily available online.

It is also important to be aware that only limited studies have been published on the pediatric population. These include the Devinsky[7] and GW Pharmaceuticals studies currently under way. These CBD studies are being held in a pharmaceutical setting only, and for specific disorders only.

It is true that cannabis use in general is not advisable when it comes to the young, developing brains of children and young adults. *Medical cannabis,* however, is only given to a special population of children where the benefits outweigh the risks, or where the risks *by the nature of the child's life-limiting or life-threatening disorder* are negligible.

Special considerations for compassionate end-of-life care

We as a society are slowly changing the way we die, and the way we accompany children towards death. We can *demand* more than the masking of symptoms through anesthesia and sedation. We can demand better quality of life. Our children have the right to *live* their lives, conscious and aware, in as little pain as possible, and make their own indelible marks and memories onto the giant human tapestry that holds their families - and all of humanity - together.

The face of palliative and hospice care has changed a lot in the last decades. Many people, including children, choose to pass away at home rather than in a hospital or hospice setting. As painful as it is, the medical cannabis use in pediatrics debate has opened up a crucial conversation that has the potential to reduce the suffering of thousands of children at the end of life, while increasing the quality of the life they have remaining.

Parents of children with terminal illnesses such pediatric cancers have been turning to medical cannabis for relief of symptoms for some time now in states

7   Dr. Orrin Devinsky, Department of Neurology, NYU Langone School of Medicine: Dr. Devinsky has been studying cannabidiol in children with epilepsy.

where it has been legal or, in some cases, have been striking out on their own on the black market in the hope of alleviating their children's suffering and bettering their lives.

Properly prepared and properly administered preparations of THC and CBD, usually THC-dominant, can be beneficial to some of these children. Because children tend to metabolize THC faster than adults, the amount of THC administered to them, relative to body size, tends to be larger than what is administered to adults. This does not mean that children end up, to use common parlance, *high*. On the contrary. The goal is to balance medication dosage to alleviate symptoms in their patients.

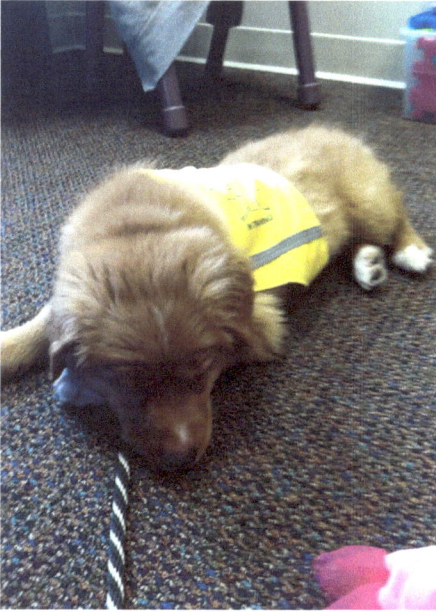

Illustration 4: A young therapy puppy in training waits for his turn to interact with young patients at a children's hospital clinic. Thinking outside the box in palliative care benefits patients, caregivers, physicians and staff. (Photo used with permission from the trainer.)

While some physicians and politicians remain lukewarm if not completely cold at the notion of administering mind-altering THC to pediatric patients, some have embraced the idea for its low side-effect profile and its results, especially when compared to medicines such as benzodiazepines and opiates. In children with intractable seizures, nausea, chronic wasting, pain and spasms caused by these illnesses and disorders, medical cannabis may become an option to explore with palliative care and hospice specialists.

Palliative care specialists, weighing the side-effects of medical cannabis against those of commonly used opiate drugs such as morphine, are eager to consider medical cannabis as an option for their young patients now.

It is tempting to want to believe in medical cannabis as a *cure* for some of these devastating, terminal pediatric illnesses. So far, no study has *proven* any curative effect. However, a lot of recent scientific evidence supports the fact that medical cannabis provides patients with alleviation of common symptom and *treatment side-effect* complaints. For these reasons, and for general quality of life issues, given the relative low side-effect profile, it may be worth giving it a try. Keep an eye out for studies, as we are seeing a shift from old rat and mouse studies towards human studies. Be aware that research in pediatrics will always lag behind the rest.

This segment of the pediatric population and their families are particularly vulnerable to exploitation by unscrupulous snake oil salesmen who want to capitalize on desperation and need for hope. Physicians and parents both need to be acutely aware that promises of cures and miracles are dangerous, especially if we let them guide us in treatment options.

Pragmatism is a tall order, no matter how you slice it, when hope is all that's left.

This said, it's also important to remember that just because cannabis as a medicine might have been unscrupulously represented by some in the past as a *cure*, we shouldn't dismiss the inherent value of the medication itself. This is especially true in the fields of pediatric oncology and neurology, where patients with intractable disorders may have the most to gain.

Take life one day at a time. First do no harm. Keep your head above water and remember that *you are not alone.* Take the time to step back, and breathe. Take care of you. Talk with your child's palliative care team members, and your dispensary's medical director. Align yourself with like-minded persons who share your goals of bettering your child's quality of life. There is a close-knit community out there of people and professionals who will help you. Whatever you do, don't martyr yourself for the cause: your child needs you sane and whole, and self-care goes a long way to assuring your child's quality of life in the short and longer term. Don't rush to decisions or conclusions.

Special considerations for intractable pain in pediatrics

The treatment of pain in pediatrics remains a subject that physicians, researchers and politicians would often rather dodge than face. Little is understood about the treatment of pain in children, and *few drugs or treatments for intractable pain in children are actually approved by the Federal Drug Administration* (FDA). The reason for this is simple: the long-term effects of heavy-hitting opiates and other such medications on the pediatric population are not well understood, and it is an ethical impossibility to run comprehensive blinded trials on the subject.

The Mayo Clinic considers medical cannabis to be a relatively well-researched drug for the treatment of intractable pain. There is no reason to believe that it isn't effective for the pediatric population, too. The treatment of these children requires the use of CBD and THC in varying concentrations.

Children suffering from the following conditions, for example, may benefit from medical cannabis – whether it be because their pain is currently intractable, or because the side-effects they are experiencing from traditional pharmaceuticals is severely impacting their quality of life. This list is by no means exhaustive, but demonstrates that listing one or two diagnoses, as a way of forming policies, is an easy way to accidentally exclude suffering children with rare or orphaned disorders that lack voices, activists or organizations.

- rheumatoid arthritis
- sickle cell anemia
- cancer[8]
- muscular dystrophy
- cystic fibrosis
- scleroderma

8   In some states, *cancer pain* is a qualifying condition in its own right. This said, some impose a life-expectancy limit, where only patients with a life-expectancy of under a year qualify for access to medical cannabis.

- epidermolysis bullosa
- osteogenesis imperfecta
- severe burns
- traumatic brain injuries
- damage or dysfunction within the peripheral and central nervous systems
- Behçet's disease
- Ehlers Danlos syndrome
- Jackson-Weiss syndrome
- Loeys-Dietz syndrome
- Marfan syndrome
- mitochondrial diseases
- Pfeiffer syndrome
- systemic mastocytosis
- phantom limb syndrome
- harlequin ichthyosis and related conditions
- achondroplasia
- connective tissue disorders
- inflammatory bowel disease
- trigeminal neuralgia
- Osgood-Schlatter syndrome
- fibrodysplasia ossificans progressiva
- Legg-Calve-Perthes disease
- avascular necrosis
- slipped capital femoral epiphysis
- severe scoliosis
- ankylosing spondylitis
- Erb-Duchenne palsy

It is important to address the fear of addiction and mental impairment due to cannabis use in children and adolescents, as it is something that specialists do worry about. While it's true that studies have shown an increased risk of behavioral issues in teenagers who begin smoking marijuana in adolescence, it's rather disingenuous to compare a normally functioning teenager to a dramatically ill child taking multiple medications just to be able to function.

The treatment of pain is woven into the right to health, and the right to healthcare. Surprisingly, it has yet to be explicitly and officially recognized as a human right. In 1989, the UN's Convention on the Rights of the Child (CRC) stated that it is "the right of the child to the enjoyment of the highest attainable standard of health and to the facilities for the treatment of illness and rehabilitation of health".

While no explicit mention was made of pain management in children in the CRC, the UN's *Human Rights and Legal Status of the Rights to Pain Treatment within the Right to Health* statement (2015), as part of their Pain Initiative project, makes the following important statement:

> *As pain and suffering present one of the greatest tyrannies of mankind, society should do its utmost to use any means available through current scientific knowledge to avoid suffering, and to provide human beings with all available and possible means of curing their pain, or ameliorating it, thus granting them compassionate relief and dignity both in life and in dying.*

Special considerations for your child's neuropalliative care specialists and their sanity.

Your child's specialists have *seen things*. They may have spent long days and nights in the PICU and the NICU, fighting monsters no one could see, with a science that's still in its infancy.

Allow the author a moment of digression, if you please: neurology, on a good day, involves 50% science, and 50% sorcery. Specialists in the field are amongst the brightest and the fiercest when it comes to defending their patients' right to life without pain and life without troublesome symptoms. They do, however, recognize the limitations of the science. *There is so much about the brain that we don't understand, and so much we still have to learn.*

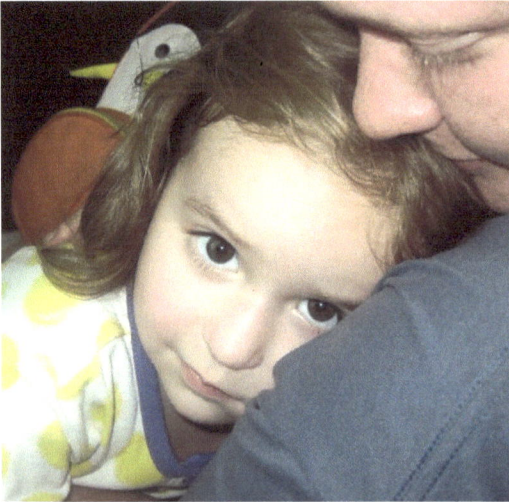

Illustration 5: E.G., one of Minnesota's first certified medical cannabis patients. Now 7, she has been one of medical cannabis' super-responder success stories. (Photo used with permission from the family.)

While a coworker in orthopedics can *fix* and *rebuild,* a colleague in plastic surgery can *reconstruct,* and an associate in cardiology can *patch* and downright *replace via transplant,* your child's neurologist and neuropalliative care specialist are left in charge of an incredibly fragile and irreplaceable part of your child that holds, deep within it, the key to *what makes your child who he or she is.*

While others fix, patch, and replace, your child's neurology specialists are trying their best to salvage and maintain, to preserve the essence of who your child is, with whatever tools are at their disposal, while minimizing the damage if at all possible. Tools are limited - when there is no *fix,* surgical or otherwise, medications are the only tool in the toolbox, and medications have to be micromanaged.

Your child's specialists don't want you to fall into the Great Panacea Trap. They are afraid you will take your child off his other medications, or disregard conventional pharmaceuticals, that you'll discount the immutable and permanent characteristics of your child's condition, disorder, or genetics, and that you'll lose sight of *reality*.

In general, healthcare providers who deal with these medically fragile children have remained open to new treatments as long as they are shown to *improve the quality of life of their patients*, and approached with an appropriate amount of pragmatism as to not *endanger the life of their patient* while on a quest for a panacean white whale.

Specialists are concerned because there are precious few studies backing the effectiveness of medical cannabis – there's only anecdotal evidence.

Your child's specialist is desperately awaiting published studies in peer-reviewed journals. There have been some, only not enough. It's not their fault: it's still practically illegal to study cannabis without jumping through highly restrictive federal hoops. What we did know about medical cannabis, until recently, was significantly outdated. We're still relying heavily on animal models and anecdotal data.

Your child's specialists aren't hesitating out of arrogance. They're being protective of your child. *That's their job.* You may think they're being stubborn jerks, but they're being cautious[9].

Bring them a cautious plan. Bring them thoughtful reasons, and a thought-out protocol. Make them part of the decision process. Your child's specialists should be your allies in this journey. They can be a powerful tool against *confirmation bias* as long as they can be honest enough with themselves, and you, to realize that they are just as prone to cognitive biases as anyone else.

---

9 There are those, of course, who remain immovable when it comes to medical cannabis, and who won't hear of it. They're harder to convince. Many of these doctors are of an age where the "war on drugs" was drilled so hard into them that they can't see the forest for the trees. Bring them evidence, and ask them what they have to lose by letting your child try. Arrange for them to talk to your local manufacturer's medical director, specifically about your child's case.

> *In psychology and cognitive science, **confirmation bias** (or **confirmatory bias**) is a tendency to search for or interpret information in a way that confirms one's preconceptions. In research, this leads to statistical errors, as we're prone to interpreting what we observe in a way that supports our preconceived ideas.*

Some specialists are worried about the legal implications of recommending or certifying patients for cannabis registries. Some healthcare professionals are still leery of federal authorities and licensure implications of recommending and documenting the use of a Schedule 1 substance in a patient, let alone doing it with a pediatric patient. There are federal laws in place protecting physicians against federal retaliation, and an amendment was passed in the Spring of 2015 preventing federal funds from being used to actively chase down and sue individuals for federal crimes related to cannabis use in states where it is legal (including for medical purposes). This offers more protection than ever before, but still, who wants to get sued?

In this uncertain environment, some physicians are understandably nervous. Some must also bow to the decisions made by their hospitals, clinics and umbrella organizations who may have created policies against certification of patients[10] under some or all circumstances.

Physicians have concerns about their patients finding themselves without access to their medicines should they become hospitalized, as some hospitals have policies against the use of cannabis in their facilities or on their grounds.

---

10 Because cannabis is, federally, a Schedule 1 substance, medical doctors cannot *prescribe* it. They can *certify* that a certain patient has a medical condition that qualifies them for registration into a state's medical cannabis program. Doctors have no control over what their patients are actually dispensed: they can only certify that their patient has a qualifying condition under the state's laws. They can, of course, make recommendations based on their understanding of the current research and their knowledge of your child's condition(s).

This is a valid concern, and one you need to consider before heading down this path, especially if your child is using cannabis as the dominant medication (or the only medication) to treat his or her medical condition.

Some medical associations, hospital groups, and other professional associations may have issued policy statements that could put your child's doctor's job at risk.

These are all important questions, and important issues. The best course of action is to treat the problem with a level-headed approach, and to open the discussion with your child's practitioner as one would regarding any *new experimental treatment.*

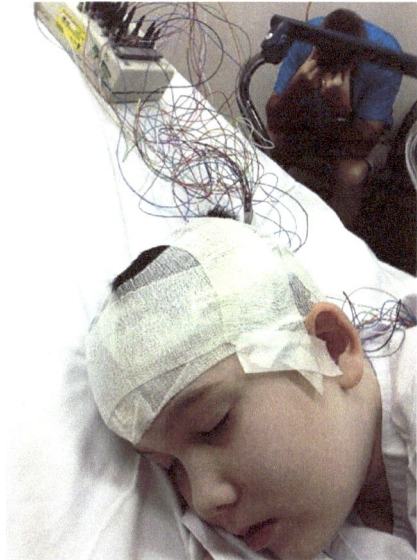

❊

Illustration 6: J.W., an Australian boy diagnosed with a complex, catastrophic set of childhood epilepsy syndromes undergoes an EEG while his distraught father watches over him. Since starting treatment with medical cannabis, J.W. has made remarkable progress and is almost seizure-free. His parents continue to fight for legal access to medical cannabis in Australia.

❦ II ❧

Medical Cannabis 101: The Basics

Cannabis, by any other name, smells as sweet? Or, really, as awful?

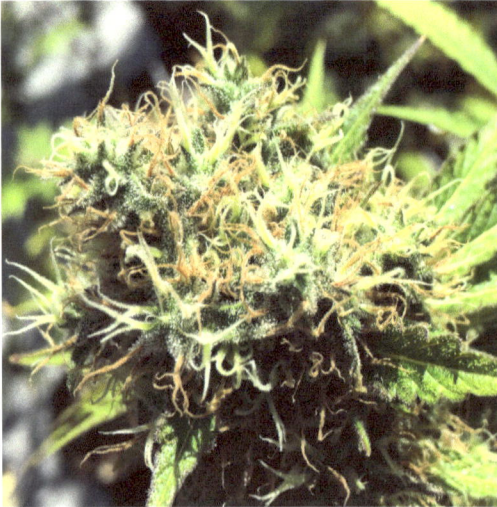

Illustration 7: Flower of a female cannabis sativa plant.
Photo credit: Vireo Health (2015)

Yes. It kind of does. Cannabis, marijuana, hemp – all refer to the same family of plants. How we classify them, and how we legally treat them (or don't) has a sordid, bizarre prohibitionist history.

Here's the story, without getting into the more complex details (which you're welcome to go dive into, there are plenty of wonderful technical manuals to help you do just that).

Man has been cultivating cannabis plants since the beginning of time – or, at least, since the beginning of his forays into agriculture in south and central Asia. Hemp spread quickly from one continent to the other: its seeds are nutritious, the plants make for a relatively hearty crop and its fibers could be used for making incredibly strong rope, sturdy textiles, paper, and *medicine.*

There are three separate species of the plant – one which is small and rather atypical, localized to Eastern Europe and Russia – and two with which we are most familiar: *Cannabis sativa* (which is tall and lanky, and often associated with THC) and *Cannabis indica* (which is rather short, squat, quicker to flower and associated with industrial applications such as hemp and hemp oils, and tends to contain more CBD).

When the plant flowers, its trichomes[11] produce a resin that contains concentrated psychoactive[12] substances, notably THC (tetrahydrocannabinol). But here's the deal: Cannabis sativa and indica contain at least eighty-five cannabinoids, many of which have some medicinal significance, and some of which we're barely starting to understand.

What varies are the concentrations (or percentages) of these cannabinoids depending on the species or hybrid being grown by cultivators. Some cultivators grow cannabis for its THC, others for its CBD, some for its textile strength, some for various medicinal or even spiritual properties. Properties vary by species, by strain, by individual *plant* - partly by genetics, and partly by cultivation method, too.

Some laws allow for the growing of *industrial hemp*, which by legal definition only includes cannabis that contains less than 0.3% THC by dry weight. An example of such a plant is the notorious *Charlotte's Web*, which started its life as a cannabis sativa plant named "The Hippie's Disappointment[13]", but stands to be reclassified as *industrial hemp* after generations of selective breeding. You can see why it becomes hard to produce medicine that is *consistent* when you're

---

11 *small hairs or outgrowths*

12 *'affecting the mind', or in common parlance, 'mind-altering'.*

13 *The Hippie's Disappointment* is devoid of almost all THC, making it an essentially non-psychoactive plant. If ingested or smoked, someone looking to get high would, in fact, be quite disappointed.

dealing with a naturally inconsistent design - as all plants are. While it is popular to name strains of cannabis plants, it is the *active ingredients contained therein* that truly count. In the end, the testable cannabinoid content is what matters to patients. This is where science and nature meet, and it's a beautiful thing.

When we treat patients with *medical cannabis*, we usually treat them with *specific cannabinoids or combinations of those specific cannabinoids* (making use of a phenomenon called *the entourage effect* - more on that later) rather than trying to hammer a nail into a deck with a steam roller. Manufacturers of oils and tinctures make medications to specifications to isolate cannabinoids they want and need, to the benefit of their patients.

This is a somewhat controversial practice in the recreational user world, but it remains a scientifically sound practice: it allows us to isolate moving parts, and figure out what components are acting upon what, with measurable data. Most focus on the two main cannabinoids (THC and CBD) in their patient literature to keep things simpler for people to understand, but those are not the only cannabinoids involved in their products.

Wait, you mean they split up the plant stuffs, and put them back together again? I thought medical cannabis was "all natural"!

Medical cannabis is *all natural* in that it is extracted from plants. Picture a long-haired farmer watching over his cannabis crop, silently praying for the people whose lives he will save, at no cost other than his sweat, tears, and the occasional bundle of kale. Many think that *this romanticized illusion* is what the medical cannabis industry should be about. But there's more to it than *farm to table, oil to face*.

Comical image aside, part of it is true: it *is* a labor of love, but it is also an industry that requires expensive machinery, clinical precision, and an inordinate amount of attention to detail if this process is to be done right. The science behind extracting the cannabinoids from the cannabis plants and producing a reliable, consistent, measurable, *replicable and safe* product is complex and incredibly expensive, but it is vitally important. While some patients may not be particularly sensitive to fluctuations in cannabinoid contents and concentrations, children appear to be. Making medications that are deconstructed and reconstructed with precision and care can make the difference between a product that is uniform and remains the same, and a child who experiences a sudden loss of medicine efficacy and lands in the ER in status epilepticus, or an immunocompromised child who suddenly sprouts a fungal infection. There are also unnecessary leftover natural components, such as chlorophyll and wax, that are not the type of substances that are all that great to have contained in children's medicine.

Whole plant products do benefit some patients. In pediatric epilepsies and other complex medical conditions involving *medically fragile children*, the ability to replicate medication with precision and consistency is proving to be helpful and may pave the way to better research and greater cooperation in research. The more variables can be controlled, the less doubt is created, and the more reliable the results, the more value anecdotal data has to researchers.

What are the cannabinoids and what do they do?

Cannabinoids are a class of chemical compounds that act on cannabinoid receptors in cells that repress neurotransmitter release in the brain. They are not solely found in cannabis plants, but don't appear in other plants in a significant amount. The most notable cannabinoid is the phytocannabinoid tetrahydrocannabinol (THC). Cannabidiol (CBD) is the major cannabinoid people associate with the treatment of refractory epilepsies[14].

---

14 *refractory epilepsy* is defined as a seizure disorder that has the infuriating tendency to be resistant (or quite literally *unyielding*) to treatment. The word comes from the Latin *refractarius,* meaning *stubborn.*

THC	Tetrahydrocannabinol	The best known cannabinoid, and the primary psychoactive compound of cannabis. It has neuroprotective and analgesic effects, too. Often used in cancer, pain, and in the treatment of intractable nausea.
CBD	Cannabidiol	CBD is a non-psychoactive cannabinoid that has shown great promise in the treatment of refractory epilepsies. Numerous medical benefits have been attributed to it, including neuroprotective and anti-inflammatory properties.
THCV	Tetrahydrocannabivarin	Thought to be an appetite suppressant. It may be helpful in treating metabolic disorders, including diabetes.
CBC	Cannabichromene	Still one of the least understood, but possibly a very useful cannabinoid. It may stimulate bone growth, and help inhibit pain and inflammation.
CBDV	Cannabidivarin	CBDV is CBD's little cousin, and though relatively un-researched until now, it may prove helpful in treating epilepsy.
CBN	Cannabinol	Non psychoactive, with sedative effects. It is found in small quantities as a breakdown product from the natural aging process of THC.
THCA	Tetrahydrocannabinolic Acid	The most prominent compound in fresh, undried cannabis. It doesn't have psychoactive effects, but it does have anti-inflammatory and neuroprotective effects. Some have found it helpful in the treatment of epilepsies that respond to IVIG treatment and encephalopathies that seem to have immune-related causes.
CBG	Cannabigerol	Another non-psychoactive cannabinoid. It may be responsible for fighting glaucoma symptoms and inflamed bowels. It has been showing promise for the treatment of bacterial infections like MRSA.
CBDA	Cannabidiolic Acid	A non-psychoactive cannabinoid that may have anti-inflammatory properties. It likely has benefits for dealing with nausea and vomiting.

Table 1: Common Cannabinoids and their effects

What is decarboxylation? What's the difference between acid forms and activated forms of a cannabinoid?

In the cannabis plant, the major cannabinoids are present almost entirely in their raw, acidic form (THCA and CBDA). When heated, a chemical reaction called decarboxylation takes place – this process is sometimes referred to as *activation*. The heating process transforms the acidic cannabinoids into THC and CBD. Heating can be the result of smoking, vaporizing, baking of edibles, or through the laboratory extraction process for example.

What cannabinoids are usually used for seizure disorders?

Most children and seizure patients who have responded well to medical cannabis have done so on either high doses of CBD, or CBD combined with some measure of THC. Some patients report doing well with THCA in combination with other cannabinoids. Current drug trials are supporting a fifty percent seizure reduction in children with refractory epilepsy (Dravet Syndrome, LGS and Doose – GW Pharmaceuticals Phase II trials, under the FDA).

What cannabinoids are usually used for pain?

THC-dominant products are used in the control of pain, nausea and appetite-stimulation. Dominance implies some measure of other cannabinoids present in the medication, chiefly CBD.

How do I know what cannabinoid(s) my child should be using?

Your dispensary will be able to advise you. You may be able to find communities of parents with children affected by the same medical condition as your child who are also treating their children with a combination of conventional medications and medical cannabis.   Your child's specialist may also have other patients following similar protocols.   By pooling these resources, a plan of action for your child, tailored to his or her specific condition and needs, should be worked out with your dispensary and your child's specialist.

I've heard about the "Entourage Effect" and how you need whole plant therapy for it to be any good. What's the story?

For a long time, anecdotal data suggested that whole plant extracts were more effective in treating seizure disorders (and other medical issues) because of a synergistic effect – the "entourage effect" – in which two or more substances acting on the same system will interact. In the case of cannabinoids, scientists and botanists have long thought this interaction to be beneficial, producing a combined effect that is greater than the sum of their separate effects. As science now marches on a little more freely, evidence is mounting to support the presence of the entourage effect.   Cannabidiol inhibits the formation of THC's long-acting psychoactive metabolite, and can therefore mitigate some of the unpleasant mind-altering effects of THC. Anecdotal data seems to indicate strong support for the entourage effect. Parents of children with seizure disorders report that preparations of CBD with at least some amount of THC are more successful in treating seizures and other symptoms of neurological disorders than CBD or THC or THCA by themselves.

In the treatment of neurological disorders, we hear healthcare providers talk about *monotherapy* - the usage of only one medication to treat a condition; or adjunctive therapy - the use of two or more medications that work synergistically (together) on the same system, but in different ways.

 Basically, the same is true with different cannabinoids, and we can sometimes harness this effect to our benefit. The notion of synergy – the entourage effect – is simple in that the interaction of two or more cannabinoids produce a combined effect that is greater than the sum of their separate parts. To go back to our lock and key analogy, one cannabinoid may be the key in the lock that will open the door, but others may be mightily helpful in greasing the hinges.

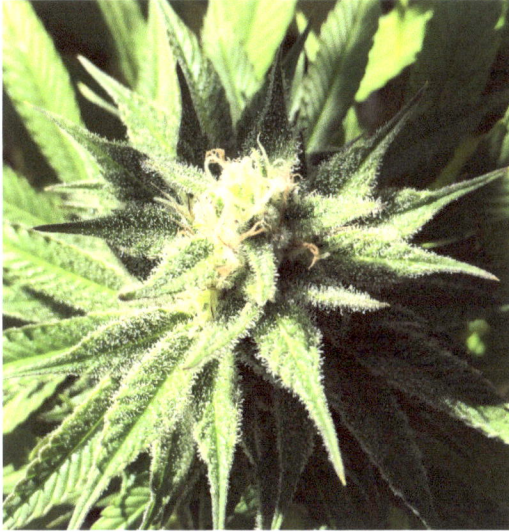

Illustration 8: Female flower from a cannabis sativa plant showing its medicine-containing trichomes.
Photo credit: Vireo Health (2015)

Some manufacturers in states where medical cannabis is now legal are looking to produce products that isolate specific cannabinoids and rejoin them in concentrations that will allow this synergy to work well for specific patient subsets, including pediatric patients, in an effort to avoid or reduce potential mind-altering side effects and other unwanted side effects. As science provides us with greater answers as to the function of these cannabinoids, parents, health care providers and manufacturers will be able to start tailoring medications for patients' specific needs and conditions.

What about side effects?

As with all things natural or pharmaceutical, there are side effects associated with the use of medical cannabis. Compared to some of the pharmaceuticals children with devastating seizure disorders have been on, they seem like small potatoes, but they are side effects nonetheless. Some of these potential side effects vary depending on the amount of THC contained in the medication your child will be using.

Patients, caregivers and parents have reported the following in informal surveys, anecdotal studies, and to providers:

- fatigue
- somnolence or sedation
- appetite changes
- dry mouth
- dry, red eyes
- dizziness
- bowel disturbances (constipation or diarrhea)

You should also be aware that some components of cannabis may interfere with:

- blood sugar – caution and careful follow-up is necessary for all diabetics and people with hypoglycemia or blood sugar-related issues. Medicine adjustments may be necessary.
- blood pressure – THC administered via inhalation may cause a short-term drop in blood pressure.
- liver function – cannabis is processed through the liver, and people with weakened liver function need to proceed with caution.
- estrogen therapy
- bleeding disorders – cannabis may alter the risk of bleeding and may require the adjustment of medications in patients with bleeding disorders.
- a number of other conditions including psychiatric conditions and addiction recovery
- negative interactions with a number of medications and natural supplements

Are there people who shouldn't use medical cannabis?

Yes. Medical cannabis preparations containing anything other than CBD should not be used during pregnancy, during breastfeeding, or in a patient with a complex history of psychiatric disorders as it can exacerbate certain conditions.

There are currently no known contraindications to the use of CBD. Be open and honest with your healthcare providers when considering medical cannabis for your child, teen, or the young adult under your care. Report adverse effects to your health care provider and to your dispensary staff.

How is medical cannabis supplied? My child won't have to smoke it, right?

Good news. No one expects children to vaporize, or smoke cannabis products. Most children with seizure disorders use CBD-dominant products, or CBD-only products. They are most often supplied as:

- ✔ tinctures
- ✔ suspensions
- ✔ pills
- ✔ transdermal products

Keep in mind that the route of administration will affect the chemical composition of the formulation of the medicine. In turn, it may also affect the rate of absorption and duration of the effects of the medicine itself.

My child can't swallow. Can he still take medical cannabis?

Yes. Medical cannabis preparations can be administered through G-tubes and J-tubes, or via mucosal membranes. Cannabis oil is not soluble in water without special chemical alteration. You cannot use usual water or saline flushes in the G-tubes to clean it out. Chemical alterations to cannabis oil for the purpose of administration via G-tube is currently being developed.

My child's on the ketogenic diet, can we add medical cannabis to what we do?

It shouldn't be a problem, but when it comes to the ketogenic diet, *don't make changes without consulting your child's neurologist and your ketogenic diet supervising dietitian first.* Preparations of medical cannabis can be taken with fats and meals without affecting their efficacy. Cannabis is fat-soluble, and usually dissolved into a fat substance such as coconut oil. Always check the excipients[15]. The medical cannabis itself is perfectly fine, but some preparations could contain other ingredients which in turn contain carbohydrates that you need to factor in.

My child is immunocompromised. Is this safe?

If your dispensary and its medicine makers follow strict quality assurance practices, then yes. The worst risk for immunocompromised children is inhalation. Be thorough, and be demanding when it comes to safeguards, laboratory testing and product quality. You have all rights to demand high standards and open, honest communication regarding those standards. Make sure your dispensary's medical director or chief pharmacist gets a chance to talk with your child's medical team leader (oncologist, hematologist, palliative care team leader, etc.) to make sure that there are no drug interactions you might want to avoid, and to make sure they are on the same page. Collaboration is an essential part of the process, especially for medically fragile children.

Make arrangements with your dispensary to pick up medication for your child without your child present as to minimize your child's exposure to other clients

---

15 An inactive substance that serves as the vehicle or medium for a drug or active substance.

in waiting areas. If there's a
need for your child to visit the
dispensary with you, make
arrangements with staff to
minimize your child's exposure
to anyone who might be ill.

*What about all those medical
cannabis pioneers I've read
about who have been making
their own preparations at
home? Can't I just do that, or
get my child's medication from
them? Some even give it out
for free!*

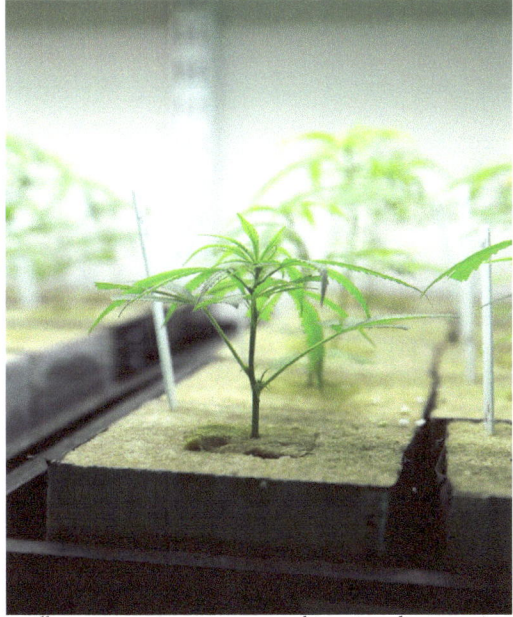

*Illustration 9: Immature cannabis sativa plant growing
in an inert medium.*
Photo credit: Vireo Health (2015)

In the United States, unless
your state specifically allows home grow, and unless you are obtaining these
products in your state, it's an illegal practice. If your state maintains a registry,
you need to follow its rules or the consequences may be stiff. You also need to
be aware that there are significant dangers associated to these preparations,
especially when it comes to quality and consistency. Laboratory testing has
shown significant issues with these hexane and butane preparations, especially
when it comes to heavy metals, fungus, pesticides, and other contaminants
picked up from the soil, never mind the lack of accuracy in concentration and
potency of the final product.

Home grow may be a possibility for some, depending on state laws. There are
pitfalls and concerns involved. While these concerns aren't as worrisome for the
adult population, we must exercise caution when dealing with pediatric
populations since it is practically impossible to dose artisanal or home
preparations accurately and consistently without access to laboratory

equipment. After preparing a batch of home-brewed cannabis oil from a home-grown plant, how does a parent know the exact concentration of CBD and THC contained in each milliliter of oil he or she will be administering to the child? Dosage becomes important when cannabis is used in conjunction with other medications. It's particularly hard when most plants are THC-dominant to begin with.

Canadian parents faced an interesting problem until recently. Oils were not available to their children (and still are not fully available), so some parents of children who were prescribed medical cannabis have been forced to prepare oils from dried leaf for their children. It's an imprecise and a less than optimal process without any way to control dosage.

I've heard you can buy CBD and hemp oil online and that it's totally legal, in all states, and for cheap, too! What's the story there?

There are tons of snake-oils available online. When tested in labs, analysis returns mostly carrier oil, with little to no CBD in it at all, much like Clark Stanley's eponymous snake oil, back in 1906, were revealed to contain nothing of note other than mineral oil.

This appears to be especially true of oils manufactured in South America with little to no oversight, and some oils prepared in the US without any third party, independent laboratory testing.

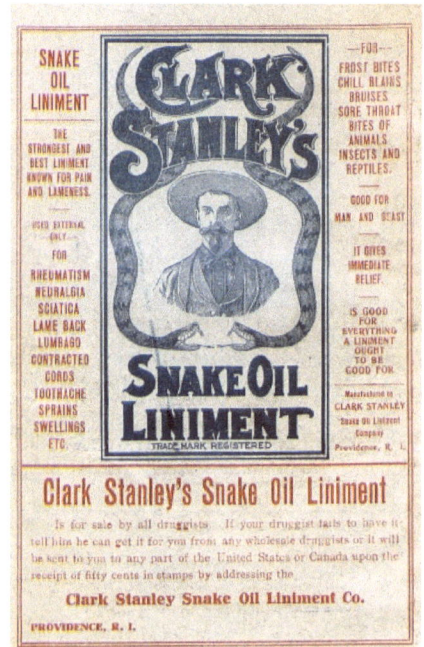

Illustration 10: Clark Stanley's Snake Oil Liniment, True Life in the Far West. 200 page pamphlet, illus., Worcester, Massachusetts, c. 1905. 23 x 14.8 cm. Public Domain.

Without accurate measurements of dosage in milligrams per milliliter, for example, it's impossible to dose a child accurately and appropriately, let alone consistently over time. Yes, there are some reputable, trusted manufacturers of cannabis oils that have been selling CBD oil as *nutritional supplements made from hemp* online, flying under the FDA radar as much as they can in order to help as many people as they are able to for now. Remember that the nutritional supplement industry has no oversight whatsoever.

When buying any medical cannabis product remember the following important chestnut: *grams of oil is not a unit of measurement.* Look for milligrams of active ingredient per milliliter – actual chemical ingredient, like CBD or THC, not *plant parts.*

Legality remains, however, black and white: no matter what plant it is sourced from, whether industrial hemp or medical cannabis, CBD is still legally attached to marijuana and, therefore, a Schedule 1, *federally* illegal substance, and cannot be transported over state lines, administered, or possessed. In other words, if you buy a CBD product online and have it shipped to your state, whether or not your state has a medical cannabis law and you are a registered patient, shipping the product over state lines is *federally illegal.*

Hemp oil itself is legal, and is usually extracted from stalk and seed. Cannabidiol (CBD), however, is not. Not all hemp oil contains CBD in detectable, worthwhile amounts. Clear as mud, right? Enter the legal twilight zone.

Yes, the costs may be higher, but by buying medical cannabis that is produced and/or approved for sale in your state, you are legally protecting yourself and your child.

Depending on how stringent your state laws are, and how demanding *you* decide to be, the extra cost can also mean a safer, more consistent product and better quality of care, long term.

If we're going to do this, what specialized supplies would I need on hand at home?

Nothing, really. Your dispensary will likely supply appropriate syringes to draw the medication from their containers.

To avoid wastage of tinctures and suspensions, parents often recommend buying specialized dispensing caps that screw onto the bottle of medicine, allowing you to flip it over and draw the medication with the bottle upside down. Depending on the size of the medicine bottle, there are press-in-bottle-adapters (also called "orifice reducers", which the author assures you is not as as painful as it sounds) which work well. If you've administered oral medications before, you've likely come across them by the dozen at your local pharmacy. Avoid droppers as they are notoriously imprecise. Carrier oil and alcohol tends to eat at the bulbs and tend to dispense inaccurately.

What about storage?

It's preferable to have tinctures and suspensions stored in amber-tinted glass, as MCT (a derivative of coconut oil often used in the preparation of tinctures and oral suspensions) tends to eat through or leach plastics. Amber-tinted glass or other opaque non-leachable materials are preferable to avoid light degeneration. Typically, this is not an issue as medication is dispensed in a 30-day supply only and are meant for use in the short term.

You may find that MCT can sometimes rub ink off syringes, making it hard to see dosage marks. Using orifice reducers and specialized dispensing bottle caps solves this problem entirely. Alternately, you may want to keep a larger number of syringes on hand at home and replace them regularly. They are easy to buy in large quantities from pharmaceutical suppliers online. Do not coat syringes in foreign substances in an attempt to protect the ink – those substances could be leached into the medicine and could also be hazardous to your child.

Plastic caps, orifice reducers and syringes *degrade* over time, especially after exposure to MCT and other agents, repeated openings/closures and repeated washings.   Replace supplies on a regular basis, check for leaks.   Don't break capsules open, and don't leave medication in vehicles where it might get hot or freeze.   Medication should always be kept out of the light, refrigerated if necessary during hot summer months, and be stored out of the reach of children in safe child-resistant packaging.

Always carry your state program card or information with you, as well as your ID if you carry medication with you.   For those using G-tubes or J-tubes, administer medical cannabis as you would any other liquid medication but be aware that it is not water-soluble.

Like many families with medically complex children, you likely have a calendar tracking the dispensing of medications on your fridge, on a clipboard, in a binder, or in your child's room.   Add your cannabis administration schedule to it.

Because your state may limit the supply you can have on hand (often up to 30 days), make sure you book your dispensary visit ahead of time so you don't run out.   Track seizure activity as you normally would.   It will be helpful to have on hand. Some families also track sleep hours and keep a behavior/mood log.

Why do you want me to treat medical cannabis like medication?

It's important to treat medical cannabis like medication.   It's tempting to treat it like food, or like a simple plant.   But it can interact with other medication and with complex organic systems.   If we want medical cannabis to be treated seriously by the medical establishment, we have to be serious in how we administer it, how we source it, how we handle it, and how we have it made for our children. Patients deserve:

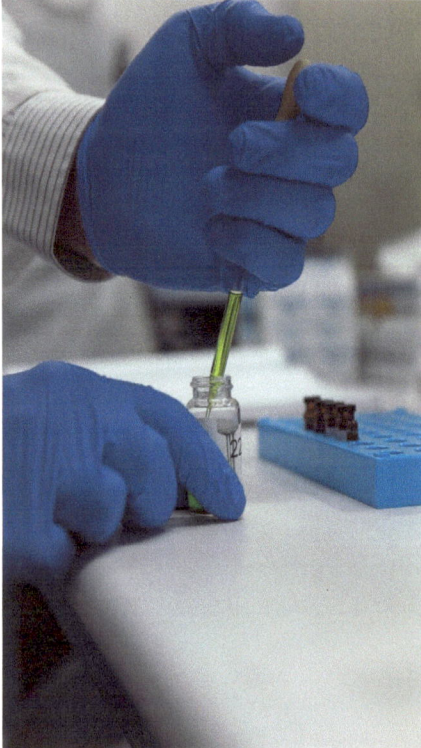

Illustration 11: Formulating an extract-based cannabis tincture.
Photo credit: Vireo Health (2015)

- ✔ high quality, pure products
- ✔ consistent, non-variable product
- ✔ consistent, non-variable supply chains
- ✔ Quality Assurance regarding contaminants such as fungus, heavy metals, and hydrocarbons
- ✔ manufacturers who label accurately and who report contents of their products back to a regulatory body
- ✔ accurate laboratory testing by a third party
- ✔ accurate in-house, in-process laboratory testing by the manufacturer
- ✔ dispensary staff who understand and can advise patients and caregivers regarding drug interactions

- ✔ distributors who are willing and able to communicate with healthcare providers, and vice versa
- ✔ lawmakers who are willing to listen and legislate accordingly
- ✔ access to funding to make medication affordable as programs ramp up and federal and state laws are being fought
- ✔ parents and caregivers who take the time to approach medical cannabis rationally and pragmatically

Also of importance: treating cannabis like medication means that it must be treated like you would *any other medication you give your child.* It needs a fair trial run. It can't be treated like a miracle-in-a-bottle. Just like with any other medication you have trialled before, it will involve a ramp-up, monitoring, and adjustments. Medical cannabis may clash with existing medications. It may or may not help. It could work well as *monotherapy* (on its own) or, more likely, *as adjunct therapy* (as a partner drug to other medications).

Cannabis components can make for powerful *partners* to some existing anti-epileptic medications, allowing doctors to lower the dosages of some drugs, letting cannabis and those drugs work in consortium and allowing children to suddenly blossom. In other words, be careful: don't throw out your child's conventional medications right off the bat. They may work in your child's favor when paired with medical cannabis.

Whether monotherapy or adjunct therapy, cannabis components could be helpful for your child, but it will take some time and cooperation to sort it out just like it did with any other medication you and your child tried out before.

When you visit medical clinics, be sure to report that your child is using medical cannabis, like you would any other medication. It may affect what other medications your doctors prescribe.

But it's a plant!

And opiates like morphine come from poppies, aspirin from willow bark, and digitalis from foxglove. Just because it's a plant doesn't mean that its products don't interact with other medications in your child's system, or interfere with other conditions your child might have.

Cannabis products, in general, have a low side-effect profile. That's part of what's so exciting and promising about them, but that doesn't mean we can throw caution to the wind. Treat cannabis with the reverence and respect you wish others would grant it, too.

This is all fine and good, but it sounds like it's going to cost an arm and a leg. Who pays for the medication?

Parents and guardians do. Because of cannabis' federal status as an illegal substance in the United States, *its cost is not covered by any insurance company or any insurance program that makes use in whole or in part of federal funding*.

This means it cannot be paid for by Medicare/Medicaid programs or Consumer Service Grants. Funds from Social Security Disability, or any federally funded state program including WIC or Cash Assistance should not be used to pay for cannabis products, as it would fall under the category of using federal money to obtain a federally illegal substance.

Medical cannabis typically cannot be paid for using credit cards, debit cards, or checks as dispensaries cannot operate financially in any way other than cash due to federal regulations and banking regulations. Your other medical supplies (syringes, bottle adaptors, and so on) are usually medical expenses that your insurers and programs will cover.

Don't be fooled into thinking that the makers of your child's medication are laughing all the way to the bank: because of cannabis' federal Schedule 1 status, their businesses are taxed at a rate that barely allows them to stay afloat unless they can shore up their profits with *recreational sales*.

Does anyone offer discounts and help?

Some manufacturers are able to provide patients with discounts based on need, income, and/or Medicare status. Others have been able to set up charities to help offset costs of *travel* to the dispensary or *support to the family* but not for buying the medication outright. Operating a federally recognized 501(c)(3) for the sole purpose of making medical cannabis available to patients would mean trampling all over the legislators' flowerbeds and peeing on their regulatory begonias. In other words, *it ain't gonna happen, Jack.*

There is no denying that going down the medical cannabis path is an expensive prospect as of the writing of this book. Manufacturers, healthcare providers, families of sick children and adults with various conditions in need of relief are counting on pioneering patients and families to band together to help offset the costs for others as state laws relax and federal laws change.

United, we stand a chance. Divided, we'll fall. It's a tough balancing act. It requires patience as we try to chew on a colossal, immovable political elephant.

Could I start a fundraiser to pay for my child's medicine?

While what follows should not be mistaken for legal advice, it should be considered a simple word of warning: proceed with caution. Fundraisers (especially those using a crowdfunding platform online) to pay for your child's medical cannabis still require you to pay taxes (a federal matter). Money is transferred electronically and through banks. Consider the implications.

Instead, consider fundraising to offset generic *medical care costs.* Talk to your lawyer before heading down this path. If a friend or a family member offers to run a fundraiser for you, make sure that a lawyer takes a good look at the operation first.

Also be aware that your child could end up being exposed to the press, social media, and all sorts of other attention. While some parents don't mind, sometimes the *children mind.* Be respectful of their feelings, too.

My child has seizures. How do I know if it's going to work?

The answer is complicated, but it's worth the trip down the rabbit hole. The hard part is defining "working".

It's easy to want medical cannabis to be a miracle cure, a magic bullet. It's unlikely that it will be. It *may*, however, make for a helpful addition to your child's current medication regimen. It may alleviate symptoms. *It is not, however, a miracle cure.*

My child needs relief. I'm at the end of my rope.

You're not alone, and you don't have to fight alone. Others are there to help you, including fellow parents, healthcare providers, and dispensary staff.

Medical cannabis may be part of the solution. It may not. Whatever you do, don't let your heart and hope run away with your sense of reason. To find out whether or not medical cannabis can help your sick child, it may take time. It *will* take patience. It may or may not work, but at least the medical risks involved are minimal. The hard part is balancing the courage to give it a try while leaving yourself open to another disappointment if it doesn't work.

※

ξ III ξ

Medical Cannabis Protocols: Before You Start

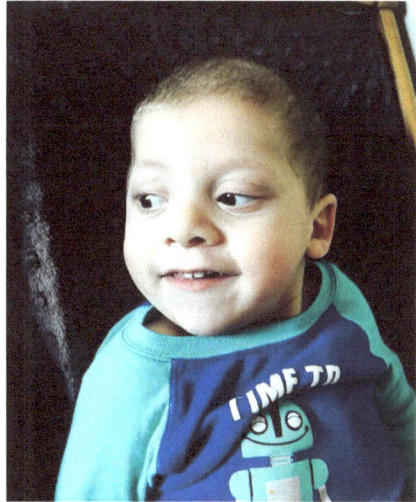

Illustration 12: W.K., one of Minnesota's
first certified medical cannabis patients,
who has been experiencing fewer seizures
and greater quality of life since starting
treatment with medical cannabis. (Photo
used with permission from the family.)

My child has seizures: Let's do this!

When someone says: "My child has seizures," it's a little like saying "My uncle Frank has heart trouble."

Seizures and *seizure disorders (epilepsy)* come in a wide variety of forms and flavors, from the benign to the degenerative, the idiopathic to those with known etiologies, the acquired to the genetic, the catastrophic to the transient. Some are caused by pediatric cancers and its treatment. Determining if the seizures are complex partial, or simple partial, tonic-clonic, myoclonic or absence seizures does little to help narrow down much. The outward appearance of a seizure doesn't tell us where the seizure originated in the brain, or why it happened.

It gets even more complex: Even within a precise diagnostic category, every patient may present with different symptoms and characteristic clusters.

For instance, some children with Landau-Kleffner Syndrome variants may respond well to IVIG and steroid burst treatment. Others do better with aggressive treatment using high dosages of benzodiazepines. Some have clinical seizures. Others don't, and only show the classic electrical status epilepticus in sleep (ESES) clinicians associate with the disorder. Some children with Dravet Syndrome have a genetic mutation or deletion in SCN1A or SCN2A. Others don't. Some may carry a mutation in closely related genes. Would cannabis work for them all to control their otherwise intractable epilepsies? *There is no way to know for sure.*

The general consensus of desperate and exhausted parents has been that if all other treatment avenues are failing, it might help, so why not give it a try? Just beware the Great Panacea Trap.

Cannabis is a medication. It's not a magical cure.

In the last few years, the bank of case studies and anecdotal data has been growing and has become more trustworthy in that the children and young adults involved have had access to quantifiable, lab-tested supplies of cannabis products. Certain epilepsies seem to respond well to medical cannabis, others less so, with room for variance.

Who does medical cannabis benefit?

We don't yet have clear-cut answers on this. We do have piles upon piles of anecdotal evidence, tradition and theory.

The Mayo Clinic has developed a rating system based on available scientific evidence for efficacy. It rates the treatment of chronic pain and multiple sclerosis as having *good scientific evidence for use* and as being well studied, especially in people who did not respond to other drugs such as narcotics. It also rates its scientific evidence in the use for pain and spasms as good.

While keeping a pragmatic outlook, the Mayo Clinic's official stance on scientific evidence for use of medical cannabis also includes studies showing benefits for improving appetite in cancer patients, patients suffering from cystic fibrosis, and patients battling AIDS. For epilepsy, they cite early studies suggesting that cannabis taken with other anti-seizure medication may lower seizure risk in people with seizures.

Also on their list of *unclear scientific evidence, but needs more research* are areas currently undergoing active research: brain injuries, dementia, epilepsy, ALS, chemotherapy side-effect treatment, Huntington's disease, eating disorders, glaucoma, neuromuscular disorders, quality of life, rheumatoid arthritis, schizophrenia, sleep disorders, atopic dermatitis, and Tourette syndrome.

It's important to note that traditional research is *lacking* entirely due to policy and the legal status of cannabis as a Schedule 1 drug in the United States and in many other countries around the world. *One should not mistake the lack of data for lack of evidence of efficacy demonstrated in trials.* Cannabis' legal status has prevented trials and research from being conducted, until very recently.

The research body is starting to grow. There's a lot of old research, lots of anecdotal data, plenty of animal models, and a handful of small studies here and there. But, take heart, there are clinical studies underway. So far, since interest in CBD has spiked with the popular Sanjay Gupta documentary series *Weed,* we have heard of children, teens and young adults with seizure disorders who make incredible turnarounds on medical cannabis, particularly with CBD-dominant preparations.

Other children have seen great benefits from preparations in 1:1 ratios of CBD to THC, or THC-dominant preparations, depending on the disease process, disorder etiology, and symptoms at hand.

Most of the children seen by medical directors in dispensary *clinical settings* have been children with:

- Dravet syndrome
- Lennox-Gastaut syndrome
- Landau-Kleffner syndrome and LKS variants
- Doose syndrome (variable results)
- traumatic brain injuries
- pediatric brain tumors
- refractory temporal lobe epilepsy
- genetic syndromes / deletions / mutations including changes in the ANKRD11 gene and SCN1A, SCN2A, SCN7A, and SCN9A gene (among others)
- intractable muscle spasms and myoclonus
- cerebral palsy
- spinal cord injuries
- intractable pain disorders

Research is underway in a number of states and countries. New protocols are being put in place, and the laws are slowly relaxing, allowing us to extend our understanding of how cannabis works beyond the anecdotal. It will take time to acquire conclusive data.

In the meantime, parents and healthcare providers can look to the anecdotal for guidance. Those currently using cannabis as part of the treatment protocol for their children can help further our understanding of its effects by documenting how their children are doing: tracking dosages, seizure activity, EEGs, overall health and wellness.

Fortunately, although controlled trials are lacking, the experience of organizations over the years is valuable to demonstrate safety data. It's important to remain pragmatic, but there's reason for hope. There is no way to predict who will respond to medical cannabis and who won't. At least, not yet.

The science is in its infancy. Fortunately, the medical risk involved with trying is minimal.

Does medical cannabis help children with seizures?

It *seems* to.

Existing research indicates an average of 50% reduction in observable seizure activity in children with intractable epilepsies.

We have all been slowly gaining awareness of the handful of children that have been dubbed *super-responders* - those who make quasi-miraculous progress on medical cannabis. These make up the *minority* of the children treated with medical cannabis, but they do make for compelling evidence for future studies, and for hope. These children are particularly responsive to high CBD and low THC medications and have seen dramatic seizure reduction, as well as global developmental gains. Note that they still do experience seizures, but until now, they had never experienced this sort of relative seizure freedom.

The vast majority of children respond modestly, comparatively. This said, even a modest response can be life-changing for children and their families. When dealing with refractory epilepsies, any drop in seizure count is considered a success by parents. It's not perfection, no, but then, nothing is. This is where it becomes important to work hand in hand with your child's healthcare provider to use medical cannabis as an adjunct medication in treating your child's epilepsy.

Simply counting seizures doesn't tell the entire story, however. We have discovered that CBD and other cannabinoids may have neuroprotective and neuroregenerative properties. Subtle and not-so-subtle changes in children's eye contact, word and pattern recognition, alertness, sleep patterns, fine and gross motor skills, and communication intent/ability is equally important and worthy of note. These details are difficult to quantify, however, and it's that quantification that medical science seeks as a measure of success.

There are children for whom medical cannabis has not been helpful as far as reducing the number of seizure they experience. The type of seizure, their etiology, the disease process, and a wide variety of factors may be involved in explaining why that is. Just like any other medication, some medications don't control certain seizure types (or underlying causes) very well.

How about children with disorders and diseases other than epilepsy?

Children with seizure disorders make up the greatest percentage of pediatric patients using medical cannabis, but they're certainly not alone. Children with intractable muscle spasms and with terminal and degenerative illnesses have seen relief of symptoms (e.g. muscle contractures and spasms, vomiting and severe chronic wasting, loss of cognitive function and alertness, sleep disruption) from using cannabis products. Treating children with medical cannabis remains controversial, but manufacturers

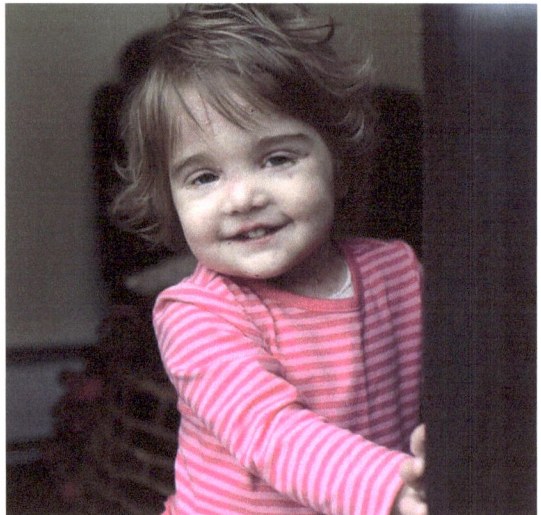

Illustration 13: E.M., a young epidermolysis bullosa patient who has been awaiting the addition of intractable pain to the list of qualifying conditions for access to medical cannabis in Minnesota. A recent recommendation has made it such that E.M. will be able to start treatment in August 2016, to the delight of her parents and treating physicians.
Photo credit: Jim Bovin, University of Minnesota Foundation. Used with permission.

remain open to the possibilities, as do palliative care health care providers who have seen its potential and its results.

Children with cancer and other terminal illnesses, or children suffering from intractable pain, may need products higher in THC than CBD, in a way that mirror their adult counterparts. Children metabolize THC faster than adults, so doses may seem comparatively large. It's important to work with your child's physician, your dispensary's Pharmacist and Medical Director to establish the right combination of cannabinoids and dosage *for your child.* What works for others might not be what works for your child. Remain cognizant of any unwanted mind-altering effects and adjusting accordingly.

There is a certain stigma associated with treating children with THC-containing products. When considering a THC product for a child, weigh the side-effect profile of other medications against that of THC and CBD products.

Make decisions based on side-effect profiles and actual risks rather than lore and perceived risk. Consider your child's quality of life. Take a look at current FDA-approved or fast-tracked pharmaceuticals containing CBD and THC, and their research involving children, including children as young as newborns[16].

How soon will I know if this is working or not?

"Working" is a tricky word. "Helping" might be more appropriate.

Beware the Great Panacea Trap. As with any other anti-epileptic drug, it might take months to work up to a helpful dose (and a working cannabinoid combination), or to find out whether or not medical cannabis is making a difference for your child. Treat medical cannabis as you would any other anti-epileptic drug, and rejoice in the fact that it has an incredibly low side-effect profile compared to what you've grown accustomed. Patience is the key. Parents from Minnesota's medical cannabis program and from online support

---

16 In the spring of 2015, the FDA approved trials for the treatment of neonatal hypoxic ischemic encephalopathy using IV CBD (GW Pharmaceuticals).

groups for registered pediatric patients from medical-legal states report a six-month window of trial and error before getting a feel for whether or not improvement is truly settling in, factoring in the "start low, go slow" ramp-up titration, and the settling time into the medication adjustment period.

When do I know it's time to give this a try?

In my experience, parents, caregivers and healthcare providers who turn to medical cannabis for their patients are out of traditional pharmaceutical options. They're often out of surgical treatment options as well. Many turn to it when entering neuropalliative care, palliative or hospice care programs.

When is it time to try new, experimental therapies? Only you and your child's treatment team know. It comes down to a quality of life issue. Does this mean you have to wait until there are no other options? Not necessarily. Patients and their caregivers should have the right to take risks and try new treatments.

How do I know it's not all the placebo effect?

Scientifically, you don't. Anecdotally, there is a lot of evidence supporting that it's not.

Hold the phone: I keep hearing this "scientific evidence" and "anecdotal evidence" distinction thing. How can scientists and doctors dismiss what they're calling anecdotal evidence like it's bad?!

Good news: They're not. In popular culture, we associate the expression *scientific evidence* with something that is *immovably true.* We think anything dubbed *anecdotal* means a *story spun out of thin air without factual supports.* This isn't universally true.

In medicine, anecdotal evidence can include non-blinded trials or case studies. These are often heavily documented, and can include reams of raw, objective metrics and data, like an EEG pre- and post- treatment with a new experimental drug. They are, however, based on individual reports, and haven't been reproduced in controlled, double-blind, large sample settings. They involved *no controls*. They help point us in directions research should go for further investigation, but they do not fully take out the human bias factors when it comes to interpreting the data extrapolated.

Scientific evidence helps us answer the question: *"Am I seeing what I think I'm seeing, and for the reasons that I think are the underlying cause?"* These are important questions to ask. Correlation, causation and coincidence are not the same thing.

As with anything that hasn't been tested in double blind studies – especially a drug like this one that is being given in such a desperate-for-relief population – we are plagued by *confirmation bias*. In other words, we want this to work so badly that we assume every little change we see as proof that it does. We assume every setback is caused by something else. Overall, the picture might not be changing at all, but we want it to so much that we think it is. Confirmation bias is hard to avoid, especially for parents. The best way to find out if cannabis itself is working for your child is to dutifully log what you see: visible seizures, changes in behavior (ask teachers and therapists to observe, as well, and report back), as well as neuropsychiatric testing and EEG results. Ask healthcare providers for their opinion.

How do we figure out dosage? My child's doctor doesn't know where to start, and besides, the law is such that he only can recommend medical cannabis, not prescribe it. What do I do?!

Every manufacturer's advice has been to *start low, go slow* (with the notable exception of GW Pharmaceuticals' FDA-approved drug trial).

For epilepsy, CBD-dominant products often start with a dose of 0.25-0.5mg of CBD per pound per day, administered in three divided doses (one morning, one midday, one evening).

Increase the dose by 0.25-0.5mg per pound every three weeks until marked improvement and an equilibrium settles in, or until a 2.0mg/pound level has been reached.

Keep in mind that these products contain THC, and that CBD-only products will require a different dosing scheme.

> ### *Example*
> Emma, a non-speaking child with intractable epilepsy, weighs 50 pounds. Her current medications include clobazam (Onfi/Frisium), valproate (Depakote/Epilim/valproic acid), and levetiracetam (Keppra).
>
> Her starting dose for a common preparation of CBD-dominant medical cannabis would be (split into two or three doses a day):
>
> > 0.25 x 50 = 12.5mg per day for the first three weeks
> > 0.50 x 50 = 25mg per day for the fourth, fifth and sixth week
> > ... and so on, until symptoms improve or goal dose is reached.
>
> For Emma, a therapeutic dose of medical cannabis, at 2.0mg of CBD per pound, *might be* 100mg of CBD every day, in divided doses. If Emma's tincture is formulated to contain 50mg of CBD per milliliter, she would take 2mL every day, in divided doses. If she takes an oral suspension through her G-tube that is formulated to contain 20mg per milliliter, she would then take 5mL per day, in divided doses, and so on.
>
> Emma's labs should be drawn and her medication levels should be checked. Her clobazam may need to be reduced, as CBD tends to make

clobazam more bioavailable. She may need less of it to see the same effects, and may appear more sedated until a better balance is reached.

Her valproate levels may also rise and should be monitored. Levetiracetam levels have been shown to rise between 15 and 50% in some patients, and should be monitored. The reason for this is not known. Rapidly changing her levetiracetam, clobazam, or valproate could lead to severe headaches, breakthrough seizures and cause her behavior to disintegrate. *Extreme caution* in weaning any of her medications is advisable.

Never attempt to wean or adjust medications without the help of your child's physician.

Start low, go slow, and keep an eye out for changes. Do not suddenly change or wean your child's other medications. Ask your child's healthcare provider for labs. Monitor serum levels closely.

For cancer, pain, and other complex conditions, protocols need to be tailored for each child and may vary widely. In these children, medical cannabis may be more heavily weighted towards THC rather than CBD, or aimed at a balance of the two.

When you make a plan for your child with your dispensary, outline the plan for the coming months, and think ahead. That way, you will get a sense of where you are headed rather than feeling like you are flying by the seat of your pants.

It is likely that you will need to readjust this plan depending on how your child is responding to medical cannabis, and if you are adjusting any other medications (or if your child happens to get sick somewhere in the middle, just to keep you on your toes). It's a nice way to help you feel grounded.

How do we know when to stop? How long do we try before giving up?

That's an excellent question. Consider what you have done with other medications in the past. In most cases, your doctor would ask for you to get your child to a *therapeutic range* first, and then give that therapeutic range a trial run of a couple of months. In general, it takes twelve weeks to ramp up medical cannabis to therapeutic range. Then, plan for a stabilization period. Then, if desired by you *and* by your child's physician, factor and plan in a medicine wean or adjustment period as well, as it may affect reaching the therapeutic range. Plan for a final stabilization period.

On the whole, this can take an average of four to six months or more to try, if you're going to give the process a fair shot. There are exceptions of course: immediate adverse reactions being the most evident one of them. Talk to your child's doctor and to your dispensary staff, and do not abruptly stop treatment.

Is there a way to test CBD drug levels?

As of the first printing of this book, no. The University of Minnesota is developing such a test in a research capacity and not yet for commercial laboratory use.

I was told my child might benefit from a higher THC dosage than what's normally used for seizure disorders. Will the THC make my child "high"?

Your child won't suddenly start calling you *dude*. You shouldn't necessarily stock up on cheesy crackers from the local warehouse club, unless they're already a staple in your house. The fact that we worry about making these critically ill children *high* with medical cannabis shows that a lot of work needs to be done to change perceptions. We're not about to be overrun by tiny stoners in light-up tennis shoes.

Your child won't get "high". With a proper balance of CBD and THC, the psychoactive effects of THC can be mitigated, while the benefits of THC – pain control, nausea and vomiting control, appetite stimulation, muscle spasm reduction – can be amplified. With a little luck and some adjustments over time, your child's sleep patterns may also improve.

Your dispensary's pharmacist or medical director will be able to best guide you, along with your child's palliative care provider, when it comes to finding the proper cannabinoid balance to bring your child the best symptom relief available with the fewest negative side effects. Always remember to aim for the best quality of life. *The rest is secondary.*

When compared to the other pharmaceuticals our children have been on – from benzodiazepines to opiates – the potential psychoactive effect of THC seems like small potatoes.

Some people say we need to administer the medical cannabis two hours before other medication. There's no way we can juggle all those meds with work, and school, and therapies. Do we have to?

The short answer is no. Compliance and consistency are more important than theoretical timing of doses.

Yes, there may be implications on absorption and processing of the cannabinoids and the other medication your child is taking, but it may work in your child's favor to take the cannabis at the same time as his or her other medication.

For example, a child with severe insomnia issues and nocturnal seizures may do well pairing the night time cannabis dose with her night time benzodiazepine as both might work well hand-in-hand. Consult your child's neurologist, your dispensary's Medical Director or Pharmacist. They will be able to help you.

Remember that what is recommended for one patient may not be the recommendation for another. Drug profiles and interactions, disease process and etiology, age and other factors all play a part in recommendations.

CBD has a long half-life, so dosing timing is less important. THC duration depends on the route of administration, but parents find that a minimum of twice a day dosing gives better effects.

Relationship to meals can be important however: medication is best absorbed with fatty meals, as cannabinoids are fat soluble. It would be best to avoid combining it with drinks like orange juice, which are water and acid.

When in doubt, ask.

What about allergies?

Cannabis is a plant that contains thousands of chemical compounds: it is possible to have an allergic reaction to one or any of these compounds. You won't know until they've been tried. There have been some anecdotal reports of people allergic to hops (which is in the Cannabinaceae family) also being allergic to cannabis.

Medical cannabis preparations also contain inactive ingredients, in order to turn raw cannabis into capsule, tincture, and oil forms. Many manufacturers use coconut oil extract (MCT) as a carrier oil.

If your child has a coconut allergy, you will need to find an alternative source. Some also use colorings and flavorings, which might trigger allergic reactions. Some manufacturers have successfully used olive oil as a carrier for small batches for their clients with allergies, but this is not common practice.

Be sure to discuss allergies with your providers. They're there to help.

Do I need to worry about contaminants, heavy metals, and harmful chemicals?

Depending on where and how plants are grown (no, growing plants "organically and outdoors" does not a safe crop make – heavy metals come from dirt), and how your medication is produced, these are things you may have to be concerned about. Being informed is critical.

For example, in Minnesota and New York, manufacturers can only use carbon dioxide (CO_2) to extract cannabinoids from the plant, which leaves no residue behind. Growing plants in a greenhouse using advanced hydroponic principles also avoids the introduction of harmful chemicals, contaminants and other harmful substances.

The most diligent manufacturers will test their products for contaminants such as pesticides and heavy metals, and will do additional quality testing throughout the processing of their plant materials to make sure they produce the safest and highest quality medicines they can. Few do both in-house testing and third-party testing, but for the sake of the safety of this particularly vulnerable patient population, more should.

Can flavorings be added to the medicine to make it more palatable?

In certain circumstances, yes. Parents often find it easier to follow up the administration of oils with a strong-tasting substance such as chocolate pudding.

What are the legal implications of starting this protocol?

This is the million dollar question, and one that people fail to ask when they probably should. When in doubt, consult an attorney who is familiar with cannabis. What follows is not, and should not be considered, legal advice. It is only meant to help you consider implications you might have not thought of, so you can inform yourself and consult the appropriate legal counsel if necessary.

Currently, cannabis is still a Schedule 1 substance, which means it is federally considered an illegal drug. Its legality varies from state to state. If you live in a state where medical cannabis is legal, you need to be aware that possession of medical cannabis and administration of medical cannabis can have an impact on the following:

- ✔ Hospital admission: Some hospitals will not allow the administration of medical cannabis or its possession on their property. This becomes important if your child has to be hospitalized, or enters an in-patient hospice care program.

- ✔ Schooling: Medical cannabis *cannot* be administered or possessed in schools or on school property, or on school busses.

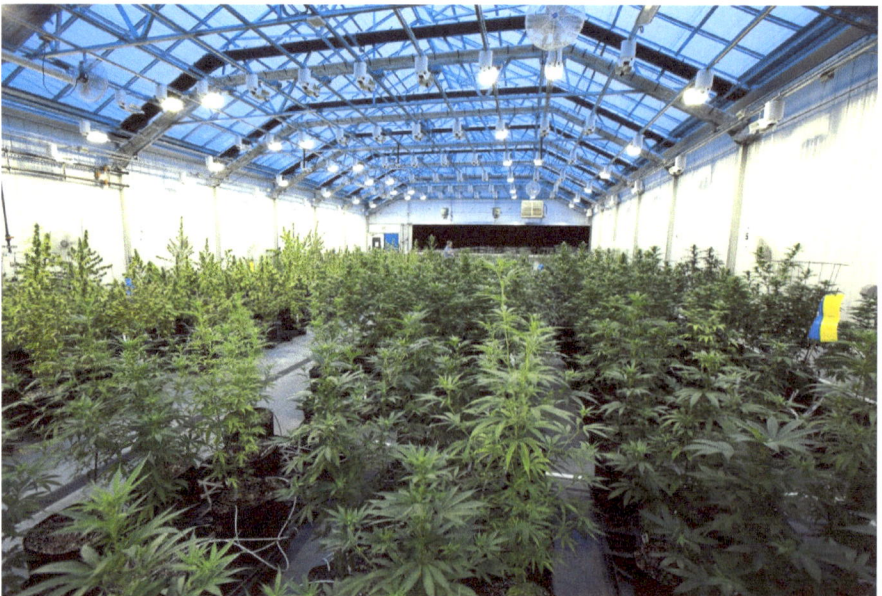

Illustration 14: Greenhouse model cannabis cultivation facility.
Photo credit: Vireo Health (2015)

✔ Possession on federal property: Possession is illegal on any federal property, including courthouses, government buildings, prisons, airports, and other such buildings.

✔ Travel: You should not travel with the medication outside state lines. You cannot travel with it by air, either. *Some* states where medical cannabis is legal will allow their dispensaries to supply certified patients from out of state through reciprocal agreements, but there are often restrictions imposed on pediatric patients.

✔ Housing: Possession of medical cannabis and use of medical cannabis on federally-sponsored housing grounds is illegal.

✔ Group Homes and Nursing Facilities: Group homes and care facilities generally ban the administration of cannabis products by their staff. If allowed to be administered on their grounds or property, it must be done by a family member or a certified caregiver. If the facility receives public or federal funding, medical cannabis may be entirely banned even if it is legally recommended to the patient.

✔ Employment: Currently, medical cannabis use is not protected against discrimination by employers. Employers who use drug screening are not required to recognize medical cannabis as a medicine.

✔ Financial Transactions: Usually, all transactions with dispensaries are made in cash, due to federal limitations on banking transactions.

✔ Insurance: You cannot use insurance, state medical assistance, or SSI benefits to pay for medical cannabis.

My child has a seizure disorder, and it's well-controlled by pharmaceuticals. I want to try cannabis because it seems like a more natural option. Should we give it a shot?

This should be up to you and your child's healthcare provider. This said, good sense dictates that if your child's seizure disorder is well-controlled, *leave well enough alone.*

Generally, physicians are reluctant to make changes to something that works for something that might not (again, beware the lure of the panacea). Seizures can be dangerous and cause permanent damage to your child's brain. If seizure management is going well, it may behoove you to let it be. Exhaust all known, researched, and tested avenues first.

As you would with any other form of treatment: *First, do no harm.* Weigh the risks and the potential benefits, with the understanding that the risk could be a complete loss of seizure control if the cannabis-derived medication fails to work for your child. Be careful not to make the mistake of expecting single-substance medication to solve everything. Humble plant origin does not a harmless substance make. Ask anyone who has ever picked up poison ivy to make a pretty bouquet.

Degree of success – and again, definition of success becomes important – hinges on the efficacy of specific cannabinoids for the underlying medical problem, and a wide range of other factors, including disease process and other medications in use.

My child's diagnosis is new. How many medications does he have to fail before we get to try medical cannabis?

These are questions that both parents *and* health care providers need to ask themselves. The answers are complex, obfuscated by matters of policy, politics, ethics and a fear of the unknown.

Patients and their proxies have a fundamental right to take risks and help direct care. While the medical cannabis discourse seems to have taken a turn for reserving use only for intractable and refractory disorders that don't respond to conventional treatment, it's worthwhile considering the value of medical cannabis for the treatment of a wide range of disorders no matter the severity.

When making *any* treatment decision, it's important to assess risks against benefits. In the treatment of seizures, for example, one should remember that a great number of anti-epileptic drugs have not been tested or approved for use in the pediatric population. Even some last-resort neurosurgeries performed on these children are not FDA-approved in pediatrics. When countering the side-

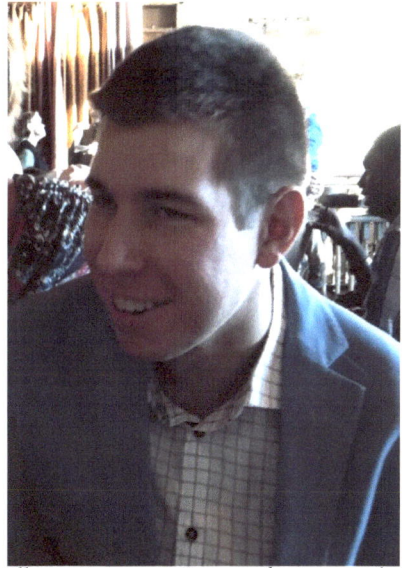

Illustration 15: A.K., one of Minnesota's first certified medical cannabis patients, who has been almost seizure-free since starting treatment with medical cannabis. A.K. had been on over 20 anti-epileptic medications previously, with little to no relief. (Photo used with permission from the family.)

effects of cancer treatment, the addition of more pharmaceuticals to mitigate these side-effects often spirals into a side-effect maelstrom that seriously affects a patient's quality of life.

When dealing with the neuropalliative, palliative, and complex medical needs population, keeping a patient-centered rather than a policy-centered approach to treatment becomes paramount to therapeutic success. It's better to cast a large therapeutic treatment net that includes non-conventional treatment, if appropriate, than to reject it outright due to policy. There will always be outliers: people who fall outside the norm, exceptions to the rules, and cases that are meant to challenge policies and force the writing of new ones.

Don't rely on algorithms to make decisions for you. Policy algorithms might promise increased efficiency and consistent application of rules, but they may do much more harm than good.

Policies are only as good as the number of lives
they improve through their existence.

✳

❧ IV ❧

Medical Cannabis Protocols: The Great Big Medication Sandbox

Is medical cannabis every other medication's best friend on the pharmaceutical playground? How does it interact with other drugs and supplements my child might be taking?

Like any medication, cannabis may interact with other pharmaceuticals in varying degrees and in varying ways.

Cytochrome P450 (CYP450) makes up a family of isozymes (enzymes that differ in amino acid sequence but catalyze the same chemical reaction) within the body responsible for the biotransformation[17] of numerous drugs including cannabinoids. Various drugs compete for metabolism at P450 and, as they do so, their levels may be affected.

It's currently thought that cannabidiol (CBD) is metabolized extensively by liver enzymes. Research indicates that CYP3A4, CYP2C9 and CYP2C19 are the likely major isoforms responsible for the metabolism of CBD and other cannabinoids in the liver.

---

17 the alteration of a substance, such as a drug, within the body.

This means that by adding cannabinoids to your child's medication regimen, existing drug levels could potentially:

     (a) spike, resulting in toxicity, or increased bioavailability;

     (b) drop, reducing their pharmacological effects, or;

     (c) cause an adverse drug reaction.

CBD is usually benign, but is a potent CYP450 inhibitor – this means that patients who are on certain medications also using the CYP450 system for metabolism may require extra caution if they are on large doses of CBD. Here's what we know as far as anti-epileptic drugs (AEDs) and their susceptibility to interactions with CBD and THC are concerned. *The generic names of medications are used in these tables as brand names may vary.*

Current evidence suggests **increased** plasma levels of the following:	Current evidence suggests **fluctuations** or **no changes** in plasma levels of the following:	Current evidence suggests **decreased** plasma level of the following:
carbamazepine •clobazam •clonazepam •valproate •felbamate zonisamide tiagabine •topiramate phenobarbital •oxcarbazepine ethosuximide	lacosamide levetiracetam pregabalin vigabatrin	•lamotrigine •rufinamide •stiripentol

Table 2: Anti-epileptic drugs (AEDs) and their susceptibility to interactions with CBD and THC

• *Some anecdotal reports and animal models suggest significant changes. Proceed with caution.*
    •*bioavailability of benzodiazepines may be affected and greater sedation may result*

Because of the lack of trials involving medical cannabis, we know little about its interference with other drugs, but we are learning more each and every day. Information changes quickly.

Parents often get bombarded with terminology that gets a little overwhelming at times. Here's a quick way to remember the basics of what the tables below mean:

Substrates:	Molecules upon which the enzymes act and catalyze chemical reactions. *It's where the metabolic party happens.*
Inducer:	A substance that binds to an enzyme and increases the enzyme's activity. *They move fast.*
Inhibitor:	A substance that binds to an enzyme and decreases the enzyme's activity. *They aren't going anywhere.*

CBD is an *inhibitor.* If other drugs are competing for these enzymes, CBD may stall the metabolizing of those drugs, making plasma levels spike as they take longer to be broken down.

Conversely, drugs that are *inducers* may cause CBD and other medication to be processed *too fast* and plasma levels to drop.

Here's a table of drugs that use the same metabolic systems as CBD and other cannabinoids. They, too, could be impacted by the introduction of cannabinoids competing for the same metabolizers.

CYP450 Metabolic Pathways and Commonly-Prescribed Medications

Substrates				
CYP2C9				
NSAIDs:	Oral Hypoglycemics:	Angiotensin II Blockers:	Others:	rosiglitazone
diclofenac	tolbutamide	losartan	celecoxib	torsemide
ibuprofen	glipizide	irbesartan	fluvastatin	valproic acid
naproxen	glyburide		phenytoin	warfarin
piroxicam				zafirlukast
CYP2C19				
PPIs:	Anti-epileptics:	Others:	cyclophosphamide	
esomeprazole	diazepam	amitriptyline	imipramine	
lansoprazole	phenytoin	carisoprodol	labetalol	
omeprazole	phenobarbitone	citalopram	proguanil	
pantoprazole		clomipramine	voriconazole	
		clopidogrel		
CYP3A4				
Macrolide antibiotics:	Immune Modulators:	Benzodiazepines:	Calcium Channel Blockers:	Others:
clarithromycin	cyclosporine	alprazolam	amlodipine	aripiprazole
erythromycin	tacrolimus	diazepam	diltiazem	boceprevir
telithromycin	sirolimus	midazolam	felodipine	buspirone
		triazolam	nifedipine	carbamazepine
			nisoldipine	fentanyl
Anti-arrhythmics:	HIV Antivirals:	PDE-5 Inhibitors:	nitrendipine	haloperidol
quinidine	indinavir	sildenafil	verapamil	imatinib
	ritonavir	tadalafil		pimozide
	saquinavir	vardenafil	HMG CoA Reductase	quinine
Antihistamines:	nevirapine		Inhibitors:	tamoxifen
astemizole			atorvastatin	telaprevir
chlorpheniramine		Prokinetics:	lovastatin	trazodone
		cisapride	simvastatin	vincristine

Table 3: CYP450 Metabolic Pathways and Commonly-Prescribed Medications: Substrates

Inhibitors		
CYP2C9		
•amiodarone efavirenz •fluconazole	isoniazid metronidazole paroxetine	sulfamethoxazole voriconazole
CYP2C19		
cimetidine esomeprazole felbamate fluoxetine fluvoxamine	isoniazid ketoconazole lansoprazole omeprazole oral contraceptives	pantoprazole ticlopidine topiramate voriconazole
CYP3A4		
•cimetidine •clarithromycin •diltiazem •erythromycin •grapefruit juice	•indinavir •itraconazole •ketoconazole •nefazodone	•nelfinavir •ritonavir •buprenorphine •verapamil

Table 4: CYP450 Metabolic Pathways and Commonly-Prescribed Medications: Inhibitors

• *A Strong inhibitor is one that causes a > 5-fold increase in the plasma AUC[18] values or more than 80% decrease in clearance.*

• *A Moderate inhibitor is one that causes a > 2-fold increase in the plasma AUC values or 50-80% decrease in clearance.*

•*A Weak inhibitor is one that causes a > 1.25-fold but < 2-fold increase in the plasma AUC values or 20-50% decrease in clearance.*

---

18 In pharmacokinetics, the *area under the curve* (AUC) is the area under the plot (brush off your calculus textbook, that's a definite integral, right there!) of plasma concentration of a drug against time. In other words, it represents the total drug exposure over time. The AUC is useful when estimating bioavailability and clearance of a drug.

Inducers		
CYP2C9		
carbamazepine	phenobarbital	St. John's Wort
nevirapine	rifampin	
CYP2C19		
efavirenz	ritonavir	St. John's Wort
rifampin		
CYP3A4		
carbamazepine	phenobarbital	rifabutin
efavirenz	phenytoin	rifampin
nevirapine	pioglitazone	St. John's Wort
		troglitazone

Table 5: CYP450 Metabolic Pathways and Commonly-Prescribed Medications: Inducers

A note on benzodiazepines:

All benzodiazepines make use of the CYP450 metabolic pathways. When it comes to benzodiazepines, assume that their side effects and their metabolism may be at odds with medical cannabis in some way or another. If you've been in the epilepsy world for a while, you know that "benzos just don't play nice". They may cause increased sedation, and their plasma levels may spike rather quickly. Proceed with caution, but with confidence and with pragmatism.

A number of patients, parents and healthcare providers have found that some benzodiazepines can make for good adjunctive treatment with medical cannabis, as in some cases, cannabis will increase the bioavailability of the benzodiazepine, thereby requiring less of it to produce the same effects. In children where sedation is a problem, or where sedation is beneficial (for sleep, for example), this may be a benefit to keep in mind. Benzodiazepines may, however, also play neuroreceptor wars with medical cannabis, in some instances. As we are still learning more, it is helpful to keep objective notes for practitioners. Don't draw conclusions from what you observe, but do observe. It is incredibly helpful to dispensary staff and to your healthcare providers, and to researchers as well. It may help others in similar situations, too.

My child takes a number of medications that were listed in those tables. What should I do?

You should talk to your child's healthcare provider, and to your dispensary's medical staff or pharmacist. They will be able to tell you if, *for your particular circumstances,* there is something to write home about. Keep in mind that all medications compete for processing and metabolizing power. Sometimes, they work synergistically. Sometimes they work at odds. That doesn't mean they can't share space by cooperating or taking turns in line to play in the great big medication sandbox.

This said, your child's doctor should be aware of possible interactions and possible effects on plasma levels, and adjust medications as necessary. New research is being published regularly on this very topic – it's a good idea to keep an ear to the ground and ask dispensary staff for updated information.

The more you keep them informed and updated on your child's current medicine regimen, the more they can keep you and your child's healthcare provider abreast of the new research and data they've come across.

After I administer a dose of medical cannabis, when can I expect it to take effect? What can I expect to see?

Absorption of medication and its effects' duration depend on the route of administration, and the formulation of the medication being taken. Some work faster, some work slower. Some cannabinoids let their effects be felt. Others work surreptitiously, like CBD.

Here are some general guidelines regarding route of administration, absorption, and duration:

Route	Time to absorption	Duration
Oral	30-60 minutes	4-6 hours or longer with extended duration of active metabolites.
Sub-lingual (mucosal)	5-15 minutes	4-6 hours or longer with extended duration of active metabolites
Inhaled	5-15 seconds	Varies, generally 2-3 hours
Transdermal	Variable based on location with blood flow	Varies
G-tube	30-60 minutes	4-6 hours or longer with extended duration of active metabolites
J-tube	15-30 minutes	4-6 hours or longer with extended duration of active metabolites

Table 6: Absorption time and duration of effects of medication, by route of administration.

Let's use an example to examine how all this terminology applies to real life in the trenches: A child takes a capsule of his cannabis-derived medication at 1pm. Within 30 to 60 minutes, the medication will be absorbed and the metabolization process will be chugging along. The duration of the medication itself is estimated to be between four to six hours, but the *active form of the medication,* which has been metabolized by the body, is still producing therapeutic effects.

❋

❧ V ❧

Medical Cannabis Protocols: Once engaged, what happens next?

It's working! Can I wean my child off her other medications now?

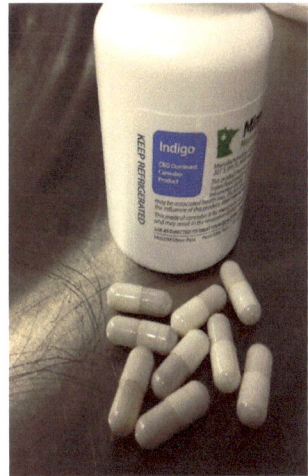

We all wish it were that simple. It's possible that you will be able to wean your child off some, or most, or all her other medications. It's also possible that you won't be able to. Cannabis doesn't work in isolation, and it's likely that it is working hand in hand with some of your child's other medications. This, in and of itself, is not a bad thing at all.

Illustration 16: CBD-dominant capsules, made in Minnesota.
Photo credit: Vireo Health (2015).

Whatever you do, do *not* start a medication weaning process or protocol without consulting your child's doctor or specialist first. The results could be disastrous.

Our healthcare provider wants to wean one of the meds, but she's not sure how it affects our cannabis ramp-up. What should we do?

There's no hard and fast rule – there have been no studies dealing with cannabis and this specific issue. The general wisdom is to change only one thing at a time.

In other words, don't make a change to the medical cannabis dosages the same week you make a change to the medication you are weaning. Alternate, or halt the cannabis ramp up until your weaning has hit its next plateau. Otherwise, it becomes difficult to tell what's causing issues if a problem crops up. *When in doubt, ask your provider.* The weaning of certain medications might make the availability of cannabinoids suddenly spike in your child's bloodstream because they are no longer competing for the same receptors and metabolizers. Fine tune the engine as necessary, but with an extra pair of eyes on the system: You might be too close to the forest to see the trees, and your *confirmation bias* may cloud your judgement. The process takes time.

So I drew meds into the syringe, and it's clear. Shouldn't the liquid be green? What gives?

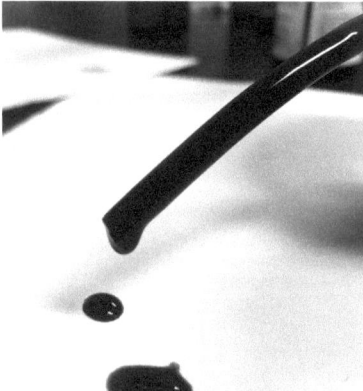

Illustration 17: A viscous CBD spray preparation of unknown ratios and provenance, with incomplete labelling and no testing information, sold online.

Photo credit: Anonymous, used with permission.

If the manufacturer uses CO_2 supercritical fluid extraction and decarboxylates ("decarbs") the product, it will remove the chlorophyll, producing a clear, tan liquid. Chlorophyll is what gives plants their green pigment.

There have been incidences of tinctures and oral suspensions of medical cannabis where manufacturers have added food dyes back into the product to give it a green or greenish-brown color. If your child is sensitive to dyes and the product appears to have such a color, ask your dispensary about it.

If the product is not decarboxylated, this may explain the color. If it is, then assume that it has been dyed to make it more pleasing to the eye that is searching for a green color. Some oils might have a faint green color, or golden color. This is often normal as well.

Good rule of thumb: If it looks like the bottom of a swamp, or like broccoli has been dissolved in a vat of acid, it's probably not quite right.

Some manufacturers out there can make CBD oils for way less money compared to those in my state. It's not fair.

Darn straight it's not fair. This isn't an open market yet, and it can't be. It's an extremely expensive proposition as it is – manufacturers who are able to produce CBD at five cents a milligram are doing so at cost and subsidizing their production through the sales of highly-taxed recreational products in states where cannabis is fully legal both medically and recreationally.

So, for now, we're stuck with what we have, if we want to do things above board and legally. We have an opportunity to help local companies grow and flourish, and help the local industry find its footing. As registries expand, so will dispensaries, and so will state programs. Trade and federal regulations will eventually relax and open up, and prices will reflect a more competitive market. It's not ideal, but it is what it is. Once more, it will take time and patience, and programs will experience significant growing pains.

We started a while ago, and my child still has breakthrough seizures. What's going on? Has the medication stopped working?

Breakthrough seizures are the bane of every seizure parent's existence. There's more at play than pharmacology when it comes to breakthrough seizures.

No matter the level of control through pharmaceuticals, anyone with an active seizure disorder is at risk of having a seizure. Certain things lower the seizure threshold, making seizures more likely to "break through" the barrier medications put up against them.

Medical factors		
illness	medication changes	skipped medication
fever	rapid medication weaning	disease progression/change
pain	medication interaction	physiological changes
poor temperature regulation	med. serum level fluctuation	tumor growth
hypoglycemia	headache /migraine	weight changes
head injury	exposure to strobe lights	vomiting
Non-medical factors and/or environmental factors		
stress	caffeine	drug use
anxiety	alcohol	exercise
lack of sleep, insomnia	emotional upset	overexertion
Seizure threshold lowering drugs		
anti-asthmatics	**hormones**	**psychostimulants**
aminophylline	insulin	amphetamines (incl. ADHD
theophylline	prednisone	medications)
	estrogen	cocaine
antibiotics		methylphenidate
isoniazid	**immunosuppressants**	phenylpropanolamine
lindane	chlorambucil	
metronidazole	cyclosporine a	**neuroleptics**
nalidixic acid		clozapine
penicillins	**local anesthetics**	phenothiazines
	bupivacaine	butyrophenones
antidepressants	procaine	
tricyclics	lidocaine	**other common drugs**
serotonin-specific agents		anticholinergics
bupropion	**narcotics**	antihistamines
	fentanyl	heavy metals
general anesthetics	meperidine	lithium
ketamine	pentazocine	mefenamic acid
	propoxyphene	oxytocin

Table 7: Common causes of breakthrough seizures.

Okay. My child had a breakthrough seizure. It sucked for everyone, but I know that they happen. What now?

If your child's epilepsy was refractory before you tried medical cannabis, breakthrough seizures likely don't feel totally alien to you. They might be, however, a source of great disappointment. If so, you need to take a step back and ask yourself why. Did you accidentally fall into the Great Panacea Trap? Take some time to be kind to yourself. Remember that medical cannabis isn't a miracle cure. If your child is doing *better* than before, you're ahead of the game.

Most children don't achieve seizure freedom. They achieve seizure *improvement*. The average seizure reduction is of approximately 50%. Meanwhile, other factors such as cognition and engagement may improve considerably. These factors are, of course, subjective. As long as there is no medical harm being done, there is no harm in subjective evaluation of quality of life.

There is no harm in renewed hope when living in what feels like a hopeless situation.

This isn't about perfection. It can't be. If this is a true breakthrough seizure, one that looks like all the others you've seen before, there is plenty to be optimistic about. This isn't uncharted territory. It's a bump in the road. You've walked this road before. Keep on walking.

Treating a child with a complex medical condition is about a great number of moving parts. Draw a parallel back to your childhood, and ask yourself all the *W Questions*.

Become a breakthrough seizure detective. *Who, what, where, when, why and how (the hairy cousin that starts with the wrong letter but ends with the right one. Just roll with it.)*

Ask:

Who?	Is there anyone around who might be able to sort it out? Anyone who might have been witness to what's been going in your child's life and who might have been seeing changes in behavior, signs of illness or signs of stress?
What?	What happened? What kind of breakthrough seizure was it? How long did it last? Did it follow the typical pattern you've seen before (this is not a bad thing at all, in fact it may well be a good thing)? Was it new (if so, should you alert your child's neurologist right away)? Was there a trigger to this event?
Where?	What's going on in the environment? Did you miss a strobe? A major sensory overload leading to a stress meltdown, leading to throwing up, leading to meds never making it into the system over lunch? Is this par for the disorder/disease course, in your experience?
When?	Did this happen at a specific time of day? Is that significant? When was the last medication dose? Was it forgotten?
Why?	Has something changed? Look at the seizure threshold list above, and look at the medication interaction tables, too. Think outside your own box, and think in terms of your child's comfort zone as well. *Has your child gained or lost weight recently?* This can affect dosing of all medication, and it's easy to miss. *Don't forget the Big Thrower of Monkey Wrenches: Puberty and hormonal changes.*
How?	What else is going on? Anything out of the ordinary? Anything different about this breakthrough from previous ones? Is this the mechanism of the underlying disease? Is this *new?* If it is new, have you written down all your notes and are you ready to call the healthcare provider to ask for input?

Table 8: Finding the cause of breakthrough seizures: Questions to ask.

When all else fails, always remember: A breakthrough seizure, or a breakthrough patch does mean a pattern is necessarily emerging. Don't stop everything cold turkey. Stop, think, and look at the whole picture.

When dealing with children with intractable seizure disorders, it's best to not think of things in terms of *seizure-free days,* but rather in terms of *seizures not experienced.* A child who has gone from 250 seizures a day to five a week has seen an incredible exponential drop in seizures. It's not seizure-freedom, but it's a new lease on life.

Things started out well, and now it feels like it's not going anywhere. I hear some parents stop medical cannabis, and start over from a lower dose, kind of like a "reset".

There is no good scientific reason to do this.

In medicine, *drug holidays* are sometimes attempted, usually under tight supervision, especially in pediatrics.

Treat cannabis like any other medicine your child takes. You wouldn't stop an anti-epileptic drug abruptly and restart it a few days later just to recapture the feeling of success you first felt when finally *something* seemed to be helping a little, right?

This is exactly what's going on with the "drug holiday" notion, with medical cannabis.

Parents and guardians are desperately hoping to recapture that elation they felt when they saw improvement when they initiated cannabis therapy. Once a certain status quo is reached, they mistakenly think the medication has *stopped working,* hoping subconsciously perhaps for a miracle cure or a continued upward trend of improvement. The illusion is a bit of a mind trick, playing on our emotions and our cognitive bias. "Resetting" has the effect of seeing a *comparative sudden improvement* often after dip in functioning (and increase in seizures in some kids) from the abrupt stop and the fluctuating blood levels in other drugs.

Remember that at some point, a status quo or stabilization point will be reached. Every child is different. Medical cannabis is more than about seizure count, it's about global quality of life and global improvement in skills of daily living, too.

If your child is taking other medication, a sudden drop in CBD or THC levels will affect the levels of their other medication and can lead to swift adverse reactions. Your best bet is to stay the course, and talk to your dispensary's medical staff.

> *Note for intractable pain: It is possible to reach a tachyphylaxis (tolerance) with THC, and require higher doses as time wears on. This is not the case for CBD, as CBD is not likely receptor mediated. It may be necessary to increase CBD dosage based on weight changes or medication changes however.*

I want to increase the dose faster – if we're going to do this, why don't we just go all out, right away? Other dispensaries increase by a whole milliliters every week, ours only by a fraction of that!

Issues of dosage and concentration are the bane of the existence of parents, providers, and educators alike.

The discrepancies between metric and imperial measurements, the dilution factors, the inconsistencies in labelling, and the downright confusing math some dispensaries engage in makes for a headache waiting to happen.

Start low, go slow. Don't go for the maximum dose per pound or kilogram right out of the gate. It's entirely possible that a smaller dose will be effective. Ratios, concentrations, milligrams per milliliter, grams per pound... it all becomes complicated, fast. You must be vigilant if you compare notes with other parents.

 You have to remember that your child's medication was prescribed for him, for his needs, and at a rate that makes sense for his diagnosis, *taking his current other medications into consideration as well.* How do you calculate the dose for your child? Well, not all medications are created alike.

Ahmed 50 pounds 1mg CBD /lb	Olivia 50 pounds 1mg CBD/lb	Jake 50 pounds 2mg CBD/lb
Oral Suspension: 1mg/mL	Tincture: 47.5mg/mL	Tincture: 50mg/mL
Ahmed takes 50mL/day in two doses	*Olivia takes 1.05mL/day in three doses*	*Jake takes 2mL/day* or Oral suspension: 1mg/mL
25mL in the morning 25mL in the evening	*0.35mL in the morning 0.35mL at lunch 0.35mL at bedtime*	*Jake takes 100mL/day* or Capsule: 50mg/cap *Jake takes 2 capsules a day, in two doses*

Table 9: CBD-Dominant dosage calculation examples

To keep yourself on track, sit down with your dispensary staff and hash out a plan for your child. Sketch out a ramp-up and stabilization plan, with the understanding that things might change depending on how your child responds to the medication.

Start low, go slow, and take your time. Chances are that your child will need a much lower dose than you'd think to reach a *status quo* in his or her quality of life improvement goals. Set goals for your child with your dispensary provider and with your child's doctor. Make these goals realistic.

Beware *cure expectations*. Remember that small improvements, where no improvement have happened before, make a world of difference for your child.

How do I know things are improving, other than my ability to count clinical seizures? I'd like to believe we've finally found something that's helping, after all this time, but I'm afraid.

There are a few ways to confirm what you're seeing. They involve bringing in third party evaluators into the mix – speech therapists, occupational therapists, physiotherapists, neuropsychiatrists, neurologists – and getting a new baseline for functioning for your child. Take a holistic approach in documenting what you consider *improvement.*

Visible seizure reduction or spasm reduction isn't the be-all and end-all. There might be other things that are improving, such as eye contact, engagement, speech, motor skills and sleep patterns. You do, however, have to be aware of your own cognitive biases.

What are these cognitive biases, and why are they important? I mean, I know my child. I know what I'm seeing. Help me out, here! Don't tell me I'm just imagining things.

Cognitive bias is something we all fall victim to at some point or another. When we make decisions or judgements, we want to believe that we are always capable of being objective and logical when the situation calls for it. The truth is that our decisions and ability to see the world clearly is riddled with errors and biases. It's a fundamental limitation on human thinking, and it's perfectly natural. Cognitive biases are caused by a wide number of factors including social pressures, emotions, attempts to simplify information processing, or even our own misunderstood or unconscious motivations.

This isn't to say that all biases are bad. In fact, it's entirely possible that our cognitive biases serve an adaptive purpose, allowing us to make snap decisions when necessary.

It's important to be aware of it, because it colors the way we view facts and how we report information. Sometimes it prevents us from seeing "the whole picture" and we can easily miss details that could be important. Or it makes us focus on unimportant details so that we miss "the big picture" because we unconsciously don't want to accept that it would disprove a firmly held belief or hope.

This works both ways: it can lead us to see things with rose-colored glasses, or to start itemizing and medicalizing every tiny twitch or behavior as pathological proof the medication isn't working *at all*.

Keeping detailed notes to report back to healthcare providers and your dispensary's staff will help a lot. Keeping track of tangible details helps, too: hours slept, countable clinical seizure numbers, EEG results, lab work, therapy testing/evaluation results, school behavioral reports, and so on.

Don't spend too much time staring at subjective minutiae. Remember that progress never follows a straight path pointing upward. It's full of ups, downs, steps forward and steps backward. Look at the journey in terms of months, not day-by-day.

Check your cognitive bias at the door: try to stay objective or, at the very least, be aware of its existence both in yourself, *and in others*.

Confirmation bias	Makes us seek out data that confirms our preconceived notions and discard potentially important data as irrelevant or trivial. Conspiracy theorists are particularly plagued by confirmation bias.
Observational selection bias	Makes us suddenly notice things we didn't notice much before, and we wrongly assume that the frequency of this "thing" has been increasing. For example, pregnant women have a tendency to start seeing other pregnant women or women with infants *everywhere around them.*
Choice-supportive bias	Makes us feel positive about the choices we make and defend them to the death, even if they have flaws. It's the bias that makes your neighbor defend his pet ferret Fluffy as the best pet ever, even though Fluffy tries to bite people's noses off if given the opportunity.
Clustering illusion	A pain of a bias for parents and researchers alike - it makes us see patterns in random events. It's the key to many gambling fallacies, and why we think that *this time* the coin will land *tails up because it's due.*
Information bias	Creates a painfully complex slope for parents and caregivers to navigate, as it causes us to seek information when it does not affect action. More information is not always better. Sometimes, it adds to confusion and prevents us from making accurate predictions.
Survivorship bias	Causes us to misjudge situations. In the case of pediatric medical cannabis use, it makes us focus on the extreme response cases ("super responder" children), and ignore those with more modest success and those for whom medical cannabis failed.

Table 10: Common forms of cognitive bias.

Now that we're doing this and that it's going well, who can administer the medical cannabis to my child?

Parents, guardians, caregivers – it may vary by state. In some states, only those registered with the state can legally carry and administer the medical cannabis to the patient. Some may require anyone other than the patient to be fingerprinted and put through a background check before being allowed to handle the medication in any way, from pick-up to administration.

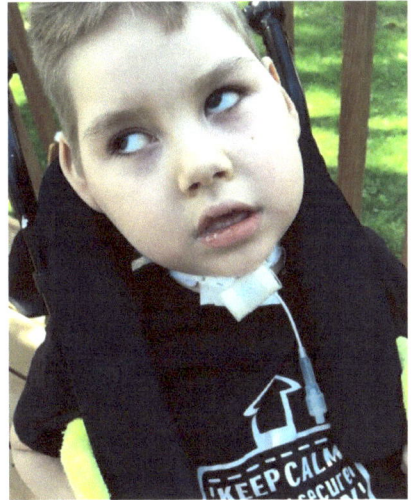

Illustration 18: J.O., one of Minnesota's medical cannabis patients, enjoying greater quality of life, increased engagement, and decrease in negative symptoms since starting treatment with medical cannabis in the summer of 2015. (Photo used with permission from the family.)

Certain hospitals may allow their staff to administer the patient's medication, but you will have to bring it from home. Others may not allow the medication on their campus at all. Some may allow it as long as it is stored in your child's hospital room, in a safe that is bolted or otherwise secured to a permanent room fixture (such as the floor or a wall).

Federal regulations are such that it's unlikely the hospital has the means to store medical cannabis in their pharmacy (doing so requires special permits, a bolted safe, and the logistics are too complex and expensive for too few patients).

If you use a nursing or PCA service, make sure that their policies allow for the administering of medical cannabis and that your staff is appropriately registered with the state if necessary. Note that if you want Grandma or Uncle Joe to administer medication, they may need to be vetted by the state and registered in the system. Your friendly neighborhood teenaged babysitter should never be allowed to administer cannabis medications to your child. Ask your dispensary's staff if you're not sure, they can advise you. Administering cannabis products to a minor can be legally a little different than helping an adult do so. Familiarize yourself with your state's statutes and laws.

Measuring medication precisely isn't always easy. Don't assume Grandma's cataracts won't get in the way of her measuring the dose right. While precision in dosage isn't a medical emergency, state limits on monthly dispensing and the cost of medication may make it a frustrating thing if not followed to the letter.

Can my child get his medical cannabis at school?

No. School nurses cannot administer, by law, as schools receive federal funding and cannabis is a Schedule 1 drug. If you want your child to receive a midday dose while at school, you will have to take him out of class, off school property, and administer the medication yourself, then return him to school. Work with your dispensary to find a dosing schedule that works around school hours.

What about a nursing facility or a group home?

Same deal as schools, universally. Because of the Schedule 1 issue, facilities will not store or administer the medication themselves. This means parents, caregivers, or holders of Power of Attorney must go to the facility multiple times a day and administer the medication themselves.

Good grief, this gets complicated fast.

Yes, it does. The best way to get to comprehensive, more relaxed federal regulations is to play above board and to be as thorough as we can be, in every legal state. By doing so, we can demonstrate how well our programs work, how well patients do, and how program "growing pains" can be overcome. It takes diligence from all parties involved – parents, manufacturers, and providers.

How much planning should go into refilling medication? Are dispensaries like pharmacies?

Dispensaries – or Patient Centers, in Minnesota– aren't like pharmacies in that they aren't open 24/7. Some may have limited hours of operation, and be open only a few days a week. Most dispensaries do not have a pharmacist on staff. None take insurance, and medical cannabis is not prescribed to your child.

The dispensary staff will review the recommendation from your child's physician, and advise you accordingly.

There is no prescription for a specific product involved, hence the usefulness of working with a dispensary with medical personnel on staff when it comes to medically fragile children with complex medical conditions.

You may have to travel long distances to get there, so careful planning is important to avoid running out of medication. Your state may also impose limits on the amount of medical cannabis you can have on hand at any given time – it is common to limit supply to 30 days, following the model used for any controlled substance. Be sure to plan ahead for renewing certification if your state requires yearly certification.

With our team, we've decided to change the cannabis product we're using for our child. How do we dispose of leftover medication?

Because medical cannabis is a controlled substance, you must return all unused product to your dispensary, state-approved disposal site or take-back program. They will dispose of it properly and legally.

You also should dispose of unused medications after your certification expires or is no longer valid.

Who should we tell about our child's medical cannabis treatment plan?

Your child's medical providers need to be aware that your child is taking medical cannabis, as it can affect other medications and treatment of your child's medical conditions. Your child's dentist should also be made aware, as dry mouth can be an issue in some patients. Oral health care will be important to monitor as it remains an unknown factor in medical cannabis treatment in pediatric palliative care.

Make sure caregivers are aware and legally able to administer medication if necessary. Hospitals admitting your child should also be made aware as soon as possible, and arrangements should be made for your child to receive his or her medication if hospital policy allows. Make an effort to remain transparent about the use of medical cannabis. Store medications in a safe place, away from the reach of children. Inform household staff and family members of what they might find, and of its legality.

What are things I can keep track of that could be useful for me, my child, our therapists, teachers, doctors, researchers, and everyone in between?

Families have found it helpful to keep an objective eye on progress children, teens and young adults make not in terms of day-by-day or even week-by-week progress, but rather in terms of three to six month blocks.

Here are things parents and providers have felt useful to keep track of:

- clinical seizure logs
- weight changes
- sleep logs
- illness logs
- medication logs
- speech therapy assessments

- occupational therapy assessments
- physical therapy assessments
- school assessments and reports
- nurse, PCA, and aide observations
- mobility and motor skills (fine and gross)
- communication skills, ability, and intent
- changes in awareness
- changes in sensory processing
- changes of social skills and behavior
- neuropsychiatric assessments
- baseline and comparative lab-work
- baseline and comparative imaging studies
- baseline and comparative EEGs and VEEGs
- the child's self-assessment, pain assessments, and general sense of well-being

Development, change, and permanent improvement don't happen on a steady slope upward: it's more akin to a saw-tooth pattern, with an upward, positive trend.

Will my child become an addict? Seriously. I was told he'd become an addict, and that later he'd be more likely to seek out hard drugs.

It's highly unlikely that your child will become *addicted* to medical cannabis or, more specifically, the cannabinoids used to treat his medical condition. *Addiction implies an active drug-seeking behavior.*

This is usually confused with the term *dependence.* Chronically ill children become medically dependent on their medication to survive. For example, countless children with catastrophic epilepsies have been *dependent* on benzodiazepines for years and their brains cannot function without them. And that is perfectly medically acceptable. In these disorders, it is *the norm.*

A medical *dependency* on cannabinoids to
control a seizure disorder, for example,
may prove to be less harmful than one on
high doses of benzodiazepines. In
children with severe pain, a *dependency*
on cannabinoids may be less harmful than
mind-altering, consciousness-robbing
painkillers.

In and of itself, cannabis is not a very
addictive substance and recent research
has shown that certain cannabinoids may
actually help in the *treatment of refractory
drug addictions.*

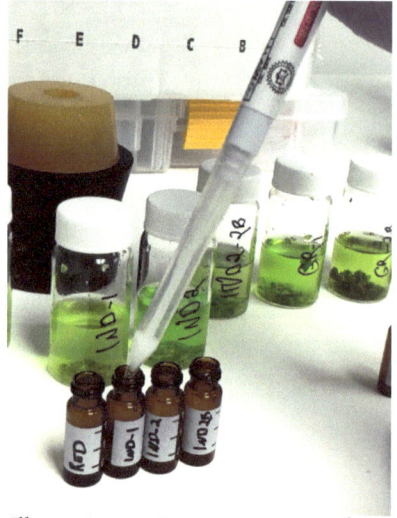

*Illustration 19: In-process testing of
medical cannabis samples.
Photo credit: Vireo Health (2015)*

No matter what, it's important to
remember, and repeat ad-nauseam:
Dependency is not the same as addiction.

**I am getting way more backlash than I thought I would. What can I do about
battling the stigma?**

You can keep educating yourself, and in turn educate others. Being factual and
non-confrontational, avoiding extremism and black-and-white thinking, and
treating medical cannabis like *any other medication* goes a long way in getting
people to understand that it is, in fact, exactly that – a medication that improves
your child's quality of life.

Replacing the image of the *stoner with the munchies* with that of chronically ill
children and adults who are bettering their quality of life will take a long time.

Semantics matter. Choose your words carefully.

The more you treat medical cannabis as medicine, the more others will, too. Helping family, friends, doctors, and the community around you learn how to best support you and your choice to go down this path is a significant commitment, but it is well worth it in the long run. Obey the rules and be a good representative of your state program. Surround yourself with fellow parents who are also on this journey.

Be careful to still run information and decisions by your healthcare provider and your dispensary before making changes, despite what other parents might be trying out. Every child is different. What works for one may not work for the other, and given the number of moving parts (and pharmaceuticals) at play in these medically fragile children, it's advisable to make sure medicine adjustments are made with care, caution, and verified data.

What should I expect when it comes to communication between my child's doctors and my dispensary?

Assuming you have agreed to share information between both parties, open communication between providers can be an invaluable asset to your child's treatment team. Encourage collaboration, if all parties are willing.

※

﴾ VI ﴿

Staying Grounded in Hopeful Times

Searching for Panacea – or her equally mythical modern-day offspring – can drive the most level-headed parents of chronically-ill or dying children to madness. Fighting monsters can turn you into a force to be reckoned with, for good or for ill. It can make you both extremely vulnerable to those who seek to take advantage of your need for hope, and a great threat to those who believe they hold all the answers.

One of the hardest parts of this journey, as parents, is keeping one's feet firmly rooted in reality. It's easy to be lured and swayed by the siren song of miracle cures and magical turnarounds. We've been bombarded by the media with articles, documentaries, blog posts, Op-Eds, interviews, and viral images of *miracles who walk among us* thanks to the benefits of medical cannabis.

Hope is a powerful drug. We want hope for our children, and we want it *now*. We'd throw ourselves into the gaping maw of the *improbable* if there is even the faint glimmer of hope of the *possible*. The truth is that hope for improvement in quality of life, for many of these children, is possible.

Problems arise when hope blends into into expectation. It's at this juncture that parents and medical professionals sometimes clash.

For medical providers, the situation is not as easy as parents and advocates want to believe it could be. Making medically sound decisions and giving advice – advice that one is *liable for* – requires thoughtful consideration. It means digging through the pile of pseudoscientific information that's out there, to sort out lore from truth. It means seeing beyond the hype and setting one's hands on new data, which takes commitment and time, neither of which are in overabundance in today's medical clinics. It also means doing all this while attempting to shake the omnipresent cloud of the "war on drugs" era.

Parents and providers can and *do* meet on common ground no matter their starting point: this is a journey towards better quality of life, and at the center of it is a child in need. While politicians, lawyers, activists, policy-makers, researchers, and snake oil salesmen battle for their territory, parents and providers are facing a reality everyone else can choose to ignore. In front of them, refusing to be ignored, are children who might see better quality of life by adding medical cannabis to current treatment. With fledgling – but clinically significant – research showing little to no medical risk, is it fair and ethical to keep these children waiting?

For *everyone* concerned – patient, parent, physician – this journey is a hero's journey.

It's a labyrinthine journey, really; one without a well-defined end, or a set of benchmarks defining success. The labyrinth could lead to the hope and the answers the hero and his party seek. Unlike Theseus, however, they have no thread to follow that will lead them to a monster they can slay *once and for all* and then follow back out again. Science hasn't mapped out the labyrinth yet, and the monsters these children fight have yet to demonstrate their fatal weaknesses.

That doesn't mean that the journey itself isn't worthwhile. It could lead to treasure (the valuable relief of symptoms), or to a key (the unlocking of new skills), or it could be that your hopeful world will end up flipped completely

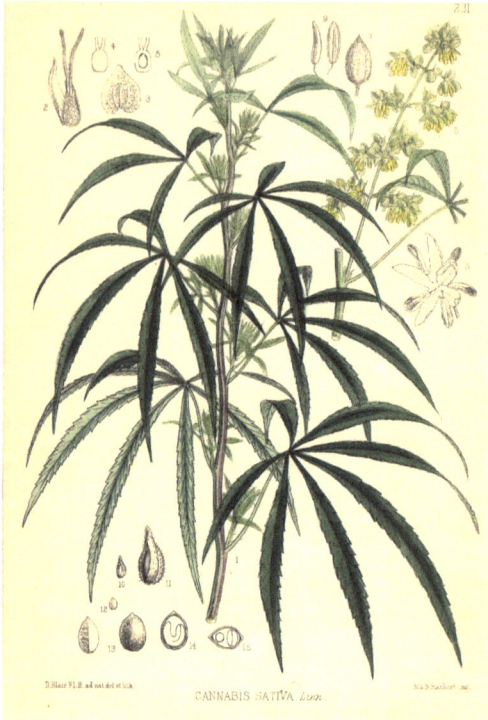

Illustration 20: "Cannabis Sativa", Linn D. Blair F.L.S. ad nat. del. et lith. M. & N. Hanhart imp., Medicinal plants, v. IV, no 231. Lithograph, color. National Library of Medicine's History of Medicine Collection. Public Domain.

upside down and you'll find yourself in free-fall; cannabis may not work, or may make an underlying condition worse. Alternately, it may lead to the discovery of a cursed chicken that you'll inexplicably feel compelled to wear as a hat (what were you thinking! Never pick up fowl in a dungeon!)

An adventure through a labyrinth doesn't follow a straight path. Chances are that you'll hit a few dead ends and have to double back a few times.

You and your hero may even stumble and fall a few times, but that's why you have your trusty party along. As long as you – and your child's healthcare provider – are aware that there are *multiple possible outcomes* to this adventure scenario, there's may be no tangible reason not to embark on the journey.

Science, so far, indicates that the labyrinth contains no harmful traps.

Many will start medical cannabis therapy and see quick, swift, amazing (albeit small, in the grand scheme of things) improvements and be elated. It's easy to become hungry for more, and more, and more, and to expect a perpetual slope upward in improvement and change. *A journey to the end of the labyrinth, where the enemy will be slain for good.* This isn't the reality of the beast.

Medical cannabis is not a panacea. It is not a miracle cure.

When the initial *honeymoon phase* fades, a certain disappointment will threaten to hover over parents. That's when we have to realize and remember that:

- Medical cannabis is a medication, which may work with varying degrees of success;
- Any improvement in quality of life, especially coming from a medication with few or without any side-effects, can be worthwhile;
- Small improvements are cumulative, and delightful;
- Only a few will be *super-responders*, but the are the ones who will get the most press;
- By staying realistic and by keeping modest expectations, you may be even more delighted and surprised;
- Bumps in the road are to be expected.

This entire journey through the labyrinth is complex, dimly-lit, and sometimes frustrating. You'll have to stop, rest, and regroup regularly. You'll have heal up, fight battles along the way, and draw personalized maps as you go along. Before you start, make sure your party is solid and varied – their skills will help you and your hero.

Remember that no hall of mirrors will fold in on itself, no abyss will stare back into you, and Dr. Faustus need not apply for a party leader position. Going down this path isn't making a deal with the devil. It's another maze to explore, in hope of bettering your hero's quality of life.

There may not be a final destination or an ultimate vanquished foe in the end, but the journey itself is of great importance.

No reason is too small to throw celebratory banquets. Don't cheat yourself out of them. Don't postpone joy.

Whether you are the parent or the physician in this scenario, be sure everyone is on the same page, and that your goal is clear: This is a quest for better quality of life. Wisdom, compassion, and courage are the three universal qualities that unite us all.

> *Keep your eyes on the journey, and feet on the ground;*
> *Wrap your hands around achievable goals, gently hold onto them,*
> *But have the wisdom, compassion and courage to know when to stop and rest.*
> *Keep allies in your pockets – you need them, and they need you*
> *To share and savor small victories together, whether permanent or transitory.*
> *Keep your heroes, and each day you share with them, at the forefront*
> *For time, much like a river flows, and cannot be bought or sold.*

⁂ ⁂ ⁂

℣ VII ℣

Quick References & Notes

Cannabinoid Cheat Sheet

This table is by no means complete, but it's a place to start. New information is being discovered every day. It behooves us all to look up new data as research gets published and reviewed.

Potential benefit	THC	THCA	THCV	CBN	CBD	CBDA	CBC	CBCA	CBG	CBGA
Analgesic	■			■	■		■			
Anti-inflammatory		■			■	■	■		■	■
Anorectic			■							
Appetite stimulant	■				■					
Antiemetic	■				■					
Intestinal anti-prokinetic					■					
Anxiolytic					■					
Antipsychotic					■					
Anti-epileptic		■*	■		■					
Antispasmodic	■			■	■					
Anti-insomnia				■						
Immunomodulatory	■				■					
Anti-diabetic			■		■					
Neuroprotective	■				■					
Anti-ischemic					■					
Anti-bacterial					■			■	■	
Anti-fungal								■	■	
Antiproliferative		■			■	■	■		■	
Bone-growth stimulant			■		■		■		■	

*anecdotal data exists, but laboratory models have yet to support.

Dosage Calculator

Common protocol for High CBD: Low THC medication (25:1 – 18:1) : 0.25mg CBD/lb to 0.5mg/lb increase every 3 weeks until symptoms improve or 2.0mg/lb is reached.

Phase (ramp-up, stabilization, adjustment)	Week(s)	CBD in mg/lb	CBD dosage x pounds	= total mg	total dispensed in mL or caps per day	per dose
e.g. ramp-up	*1-3*	*0.25mg/lb*	*0.25 mg x 48lbs*	*12mg*	*tincture 50mg/mL. 12mg/50mg/mL = 0.24mL/day*	*=0.24mL in two doses; 0.12mL per dose.*

Absorption, Duration, and Route of Administration Cheat Sheet

Route	Time to absorption	Duration
Oral	30-60 minutes	4-6 hours or longer with extended duration of active metabolites.
Sub-lingual (mucosal)	5-15 minutes	4-6 hours or longer with extended duration of active metabolites
Inhaled	5-15 seconds	Varies, generally 2-3 hours
Transdermal	Variable based on location with blood flow	Varies
G-tube	30-60 minutes	4-6 hours or longer with extended duration of active metabolites
J-tube	15-30 minutes	4-6 hours or longer with extended duration of active metabolites

Storage, Administration and Transport

DO	DO NOT
• carry your state program ID with you	• travel with your medication outside your state
• regularly replace your syringes	• fly with your medication
• check bottles and caps for leaks	• coat syringes with foreign substances
• use orifice reducers or dispensing caps	• decant medication
• keep medication in amber glass bottles	• dilute, heat, or alter medication
• keep medication out of direct sunlight	• administer medication in ways not intended
• store medication in the fridge if necessary	• administer medication on public transit
• store medication with childproof caps	• administer medication on school busses
• store medication upright if possible	• leave medication in extreme temperatures
• report adverse reactions immediately to your doctor and your dispensary staff	• leave medication in your car
	• leave medication within the reach of children
	• stop taking/administering medication without consulting your child's doctor
	• separate medication from its original packaging

References & useful sources of information

General References and Further Reading

O'Shaughnessy's: www.beyondthc.com
Erowid: www.erowid.org/plants/cannabis/cannabis.shtml
UCSF Center for Medicinal Cannabis Research: www.cmcr.ucsd.edu
Realm of Caring: www.theroc.us/research-library
High Times: www.hightimes.com
Project CBD: www.projectCBD.org
Minnesota Medical Solutions: www.minnesotamedicalsolutions.com
NORML: www.norml.org

Selected References

American College of Physicians. *Supporting Research into the Therapeutic Role of Marijuana: Position Paper.* Philadelphia, PA: American College of Physicians, 2008.

Bachmeier, C. et al. "Role of the cannabinoid system in the transit of beta-amyloid across the blood-brain barrier." *Molecular and Cellular Neuroscience,* 2013: 255-262.

Baker, D. "In silico patent searching reveals a new cannabinoid receptor." *Trends Pharmaco Sci* 1 (2006): 1-4.

Budney, AJ et al. "Review of the validity and significance of cannabis withdrawal syndrome." *Am J Psychiatry,* 2004: 1967-77.

Bultman, L and Kingsley, K. "Medical Cannabis Primer for Healthcare Professionals" Minneapolis, MN: Minnesota Medical Solutions, 2014

Carlini, EA, Mechoulam, R, and Lander, N. "Anticonvulsant activity of four oxygenated cannabidiol derivatives." *Res Commun Chem Pathol Pharmacol* 12, no 1 (1975): 1-15.

Clarke, RC and Watson, DP. "Cannabis and Natural Cannabis Medicines." In *Marijuana and the Cannabinoids*, 1-15. Totowa, NJ: Humana Press, 2007.

Fitzcharles, MA et al. "Efficacy, tolerability and safety of cannabinoid treatments in the rheumatic diseases: A systemic review of randomized controlled trials." *Arthritis Care Res*, 2015. (epub ahead of print, Nov 9).

Gable, RS. "Comparison of acute lethal toxicity of commonly abused psychoactive substances." *Addiction* 99 (2004): 686-696.

Glass et al. *"Cannabinoid Receptors in the Human Brain: A Detailed Anatomical and Quantitative Autoradiographic Study in the Fetal, Neonatal and Adult Human Brain."* Neuroscience 77 (1997): 299-318

Geffrey, AL. "Drug-drug interaction between clobazam and cannabidiol in children with refractory epilepsy." *Epilepsia*, 2015. 56(8) 1246-51.

Gertsch, J. et al. "New Natural Noncannabinoid Ligands for Cannabinoid Type-2 CB2 Receptors." *J of Receptors and Signal Transduction*, 2006: 709-727.

Gonzalez, R. "Long-term effects of adolescent-onset and persistent use of cannabis." *Proc Natl Acad Sci USA* 40 (2012): 15970-1.

Grotenhermen, F. "Cannabinoids and the Endocannabinoid System." *Cannabinoids*, 2006: 10-14.

Grotenhermen, F. ed. "Handbook of Cannabis Therapeutics: From Bench to Bedside", Binghamton, NY: Haworth Press, 2006.

Grotenhermen, F. ed. "Cannabis and Cannabinoids: Pharmacology, Toxicology, and Therapeutic Potential". Binghamton, NY: Haworth Press, 2002.

Harrison, AM. "Systematic Review of the Use of Phytochemicals for Management of Pain in Cancer Therapy." *Biomed Res Int.* 2015, (epub ahead of print Oct. 20 2015.)

Herkenham et al. "*Cannabinoid Receptor Localization in Brain.*" Proceedings of the National Academy of Sciences USA 87 (1990): 1932-36

Iannotti, FA et al. "*Nonpsychotropic plant cannabinoids, cannabidivarin (CBDV) and cannabidiol (CBD), activate and desensitize transient receptor potential vanilloid 1 (TRPV1) channels in vitro: potential for the treatment of neuronal hyperexcitability.*" ACS Chem Neurosci, 2014.

Idris, A. "The promise and dilemma of a cannabinoid therapy: Lessons from animal studies of bone disease." *Bonekey Reports,* 2012.

Jiang, R. "Identification of cytochrome p450 enzymes responsible for metabolism of cannabidiol by human liver microsomes." *Life Sci* 89 (2011): 165-70.

Katona, I. "Cannabis and Endocannabinoid Signaling in Epilepsy." *Handb Exp Pharmacol.* 2015, 231: 285-316.

Marsicano et al. "*The Endogenous Cannabinoid System Controls Extinction of Aversive Memories.*" Nature 418 (2002): 530-34.

McPartland, J and Russo, E. "Cannabis and cannabis extracts: Greater than the sum of their parts?" *J Cann Therap* 1 (2001): 103-132.

McPartland, J et al. "Are cannabidiol and delta-9-tetrahydrocannabivarin negative modulators of the endocannabinoid system? A systemic review." *Br J Pharmacol,* 2014.

McPartland, J. et al. "Cannabinoid receptors in invertebrates.", J. Evol. Biol. 19 (2006) 366–373.

Mishima, K et al. "Cannabidiol Prevents Cerebral Infarction via a Serotonergic 5-dydroxytryptamine 1a receptor-dependent mechanism." *Stroke* 36 (2005): 1071-6.

Niesink, RJ et al. "Does cannabidiol protect against adverse psychological effects of THC?" *Frontiers in Psychiatry,* 2013: 1-8.

Nutt, D. "Development of a rational scale to assess the harm of drugs of potential issue." *Lancet,* 2007: 1051.

Paolino, MC et al. "Cannabidiol as potential treatment in refractory pediatric epilepsy." *Expert Rev. Neurother,* 2015 (epub ahead of print Dec 9): 1-5.

Pertwee, RG. "The diverse CB1 and CB2 receptor pharmacology of three plant cannabinoids: delta-9-tetrahydrocannabinol, cannabidiol and delta-9-tetrahydrocannabivarin." *Br J Pharmacol,* 2008: 199-215.

Russo, E. "Cannabis to migraine treatment: The one and future prescription? A historical and scientific review." *Pain,* 1998: 3-8.

Russo, E et al. "Chronic Cannabis Use in the Compassionate Investigational New Drug Program: An Examination of Benefits and Adverse Effects of Legal Clinical Cannabis." *J Cannabis Ther,* 2002: 9.

Tramer, M et al. "Cannabinoids for control of chemotherapy induced nausea and vomiting: quantitative systemic review." *BMJ,* 2001: 16-21.

Watanabe, K. "Cytochrome p450 enzymes involved in the metabolism of
    tetrahydrocannabinols and cannabidiol by human hepatic microsomes."
    Life Sci 80 (2007): 1415-9.

Woolridge, E et al. "Cannabis Use in HIV for Pain and Other Medical
    Symptoms." *J of Pain and Symptom Management,* 2005: 385-367.

⸙ *Index* ⸙

anandamide...15, 17

arachidonic acid...15

cannabinoid receptors...15

CB1 receptors...15, 16

CB2 receptors...15, 16

definition of...14

effect on appetite..14

effect on memory..14

effect on pain modulation..14

effect on sleep..14

effect on stress response...14

endocannabinoid system, pharmacological and genetic model........14

key and lock theory...15

evidence...

anecdotal evidence..52

anecdotal evidence, definition of...58

scientific evidence...52

scientific evidence, definition of..58

tradition and theory..52

hemp..

Charlotte's Web...31

cultivation and use, history of...30

industrial..31

oil preparations sold online, implications...43

intractable pain...

addiction, fear of...24

human rights and..25

Mayo Clinic stance...23

opiates..23

About the Author

Some think the madness began with a love for garage rockets and backyard robotics, or perhaps basement experiments with recycled toasters and cannibalized microwave ovens. And they'd be right. With this occasionally explosive start in the hard sciences, Elly got her first job at the age of 13 working for the Herzberg Institute of Astrophysics, studying primordial nucleosynthesis and a lot of radio-telescope noise for the James Clerk Maxwell Telescope Group.

From there, it was turtles, all the way down.

Elly went off to study at McGill, and later landed at the University of Ottawa where she found herself enjoying warping the minds of her undergraduate and graduate students. She has since worked in a wide range of science and arts fields, earning a reputation as a passionate educator, writer, and renaissance woman. To this day, she keeps a Music and Math laboratory named the *Academy of Set Mandelbrot in the Fields*, where apprentices fellow oddballs are always welcome. Elly spends her days writing, teaching, making science and mathematics accessible to the common mortal, and otherwise writing and consulting for the television and film industry.

At dusk, she fights zombies with a formidable combination of incendiary frozen penguins, awkward sartorial choices, terrible puns, and dubious mathematical expressions.

www.ingramcontent.com/pod-product-compliance
Lightning Source LLC
Chambersburg PA
CBHW041314210326

41599CB00008B/268